Your
Childbirth
Class

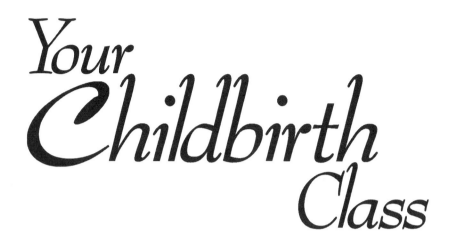

Your Childbirth Class

A Comprehensive,
Parent-Centered Guide
to Birth Options

Mary Nolan

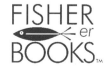

FISHER
er
BOOKS™

Publishers	Howard W. Fisher
	Bill Fisher
	Helen V. Fisher
Managing Editor	Sarah Trotta
North American Editor	Margaret Martin, Dr.P.H.
Book Production	Deanie Wood
Design	Tim McPhee
Illustrations	Jo Dennis, Pete Welford, David Fischer
Cover Design	Deanie Wood, Randy Schultz
Cover Photo	Jim Craigmyle/Masterfile

Published by Fisher Books
4239 W. Ina Road, Suite 101
Tucson, Arizona 85741
(520) 744-6110

Printed in U.S.A.
10 9 8 7 6 5 4 3 2

First published in Great Britain in 1996 as *Being Pregnant, Giving Birth*.
© 1996, 1997 by NCT Publishing Ltd.
North American edition © 1998 by Fisher Books

Photo Acknowledgments: PhotoDisc™: p. x; The Image Bank/Romilly Lockyer: p. 30; National Childbirth Trust Guide: p. 66; MIDIRS: pp. 42, 92, 116; Lupe Cunha Photography: p. 148; Michael Bassett: p. 170; Eddie Lawrence: p. 184.

Library of Congress Cataloging-in-Publication Data
Nolan, Mary, 1956–
    Your childbirth class : a comprehensie, parent-centered manual of birth options / Mary Nolan. — North American ed.
        p. cm.
    First published in Great Britain in 1996 as "Being pregnant, giving birth."
    Includes index.
    ISBN 1-55561-127-3
    1. Childbirth—Popular works.   2. Pregnancy—Popular works.
3. Labor (Obstetrics)—Popular works.   4. Obstetrics—Popular works.
5. Pregnant women—Relations with men.   I. Title.
RG652.N65   1998
618.4—dc21   98-12054
                                                      CIP

Contents

Acknowledgments

This book represents the combined efforts of a lot of people. First, I would like to thank all those prenatal educators from the National Childbirth Trust who organized focus groups so that women could talk about their pregnancies and labors, share their fears and joys, and get support and comfort from each other. I cannot praise enough the courage and insight shown by the women who participated in these groups and their generosity in allowing their thoughts and feelings to be quoted in bringing this book to life. I also want to thank my own prenatal teacher and students who commented on various aspects of the book, provided me with new material and were generally enthusiastic and encouraging. Certain individuals deserve special mention for their magnificent help and these are Elisabeth Buggins, Nikki Ford, Judy Letters, Wendy Mockridge, Morven Lawson, Vicky Baughen and NCT's two librarians, Patricia Donnithorne and Eileen Abbott. Thank you finally to my family, Peter, Sophie, Roisin and Alexandra, who put up with my short temper in the days running up to the deadline for this book to be finished!

The educators who did the research for the book are: Jeanne Langford, Val Humphreys, Nina Smith, Anna Louise Sheppherd, Jill Davidson, Margaret Short, Debbie Garrod and Elisabeth Buggins.

About the Author

Mary Nolan trained as a prenatal teacher with the National Childbirth Trust (NCT) from 1985-1987. Since then, she has prepared many women and couples for birth and parenthood. She also has worked with young people in schools, exploring with them what is involved in having a baby and attempting to minimize the fear of childbirth. Mary has talked to student nurses and midwives about the needs of women during pregnancy, in labor and after the birth of their babies. She has organized many workshops to help health professionals gain deeper insight into the support they can offer to women and their families during the child-bearing year. Mary and her partner, Peter, have three young daughters.

Contributors

Barbara Kott is president of the NCT and has 18 years' experience working with the organization as a prenatal teacher and tutor. During that time she has worked with midwives and health professionals, and has been involved in training other prenatal teachers and tutors.

Pauline Armstrong is a sociologist and has worked as a prenatal teacher and tutor for NCT for 15 years. She has many years' experience working with midwives and health professionals.

Publisher's Note

All comments and personal accounts were given to us in confidence; so, out of respect for our contributors' privacy, we have changed all names.

We have tried where possible to reproduce quotations verbatim, but where editing has been applied, the meaning of the quotation has been maintained.

Introduction

The day your baby is born will probably be one of the most important days of your life. It is an amazing experience to bring a new person into the world—an experience that will make tremendous demands on you physically and emotionally. The things that happen when you give birth will stay with you for the rest of your life. They may even influence the way in which you mother your child.

Today, professionals in the healthcare services recognize that people are more satisfied with their care and less likely to complain if professionals ask them what kind of care they want. In one way, the new approach is liberating. But it certainly puts a burden of responsibility upon us to gather information, look at the available options, and then make considered choices. It can be a little frightening. But it's also exciting, because it means that you can shape your pregnancy care to suit your own needs. You can plan for a labor that will make the birth of your baby an experience you will look back on with satisfaction.

Doctors and midwives are experts about pregnancy, labor and new babies, but they are not experts about you. What *you* want and need, what will make you feel most content in labor and after your baby is born, will be different from what any other woman wants and needs. You are the expert about you. Of course, you will want to listen to the professional advice of your doctor or midwife. But after that you can consider how what they said fits with your own understanding of what will suit you best. Making choices does not mean you are setting yourself up against health professionals. It only means that you are working in partnership with them to achieve the best outcome for you and your baby.

You can make choices about many things when you are pregnant, during your labor and after the birth of your baby. Some women choose not to make any choices. They feel they will be happiest if health professionals make all decisions for them. They prefer to give control to midwives and doctors. This is one kind of choice.

Other women want to keep control over what is happening to them. They feel frightened and belittled if health professionals decide what to do without consulting them. Women who consider that having a baby is a normal, everyday event and who sense they know more about themselves and their unborn babies than anyone else feel they have the right and the responsibility to participate in their own care. They want to be part of the decision-making team.

To the women using them, maternity services, like all big organizations, can seem to be like "care by conveyor belt." However, often all you have to do to get off the conveyor belt is speak up and *ask* for what you want. Hospital personnel may turn out to be more accommodating than you imagined they could be:

"Once we explained that we didn't want to be railroaded, I found the hospital staff to be extremely supportive. They came up with ideas before I could think of them myself. Going there was a very positive experience."

Getting information about different kinds of maternity care and learning about what will happen to you when you give birth to your baby are wonderful confidence boosters. You may feel great satisfaction knowing that you are in a good position to make decisions about your own care during pregnancy and labor because you are well informed:

"When there are choices to be made, at least I'll be well informed. I hope things go according to plan, but even if they don't, I'm confident I'll cope better than I would have if I hadn't learned as much as I did."

This book aims to give you some of the factual information you need to make informed choices. It also aims to give you an idea of what having a baby and being a new mother feels like, because choices are not made only by intellect; they're also made according to your *instinctive* understanding of what will be best for you. This book is therefore a balance between the boxes, which tell you the facts, and the main body of the text, which tells you how women experience the facts. It won't tell you what choices to make. Your choices are yours alone.

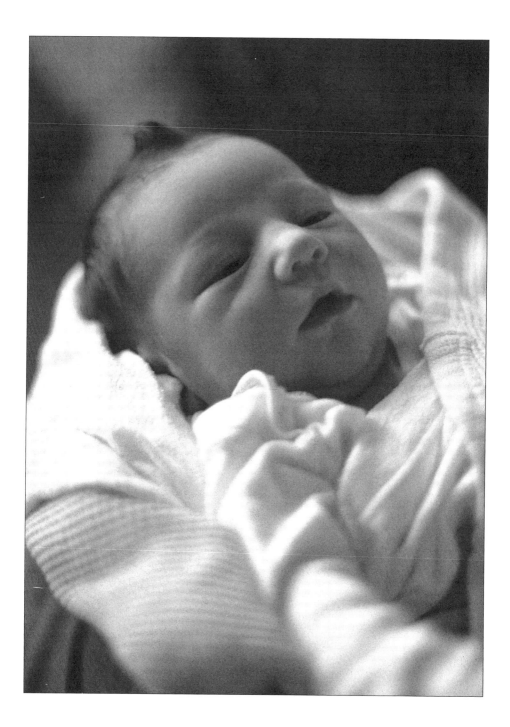

CHAPTER 1 *Pregnancy*

Finding Out

For many women, the moment they find out they are pregnant for the first time is the most exciting moment of their lives:

"Deep down I had wanted to have a baby so much. Suddenly, there I was, pregnant!"

"I was ecstatic and happy and frightened. I thought how typical it was that Doug wasn't there to tell!"

"I was told I was expecting twins when I was eight weeks pregnant. The scan showed two hearts beating. My partner was overjoyed. Right then we began wondering what sex they would be."

The new mother has a vision of all the changes and excitement of the next nine months. She thinks about many things. She'll grow bigger and the baby will start to move inside her. She'll be the center of attention at family gatherings, at work and with friends. She'll go into labor and go through the drama of giving birth. She'll hold her baby in her arms for the first time. And she'll show him off to her own mother and father and friends.

But for some women, learning they are pregnant is a surprise of another kind. It may not provoke a sense of joy. The pregnancy may not be wanted at this time, or at all. Getting used to the idea may be a slow process: *"I had mixed feelings after I found out I was pregnant. I started thinking, 'Oh my gosh, what have we done!' My husband wanted to tell everyone right away. But I wanted to keep the whole thing quiet until I was used to the idea."*

Your Childbirth Class

2

Prenatal Care Begins in Early Pregnancy

As soon as your pregnancy has been confirmed, make an appointment for your first prenatal care exam. This exam may be given by your family doctor, an obstetrician or a midwife. You will be asked to talk about your health and medical history and to have some tests.

The doctor or midwife will ask you about:

- Your general health
- Your diet
- How much you exercise
- If you smoke
- If you drink alcohol
- If you use any street drugs
- If you take any drugs prescribed by your doctor
- What kind of contraceptives you have used
- Your periods—how regular they are and when you had your last one
- Previous pregnancies and births, including abortions
- Your medical history:
  - what illnesses you have had
  - whether you have had any operations
  - whether you suffer from asthma, epilepsy or other chronic conditions
- Whether members of your close family suffer from certain diseases
- Whether any members of your family are mentally or physically disabled

Tests you will have:

- Your height may be measured
- You will be weighed
- Your blood pressure will be taken
- You will be asked to give a urine sample so that it can be tested for blood, sugar and protein

- You will have some blood taken:
  - to find out your blood type
  - to see what your hemoglobin level is (meaning, are you anemic?)
  - to find out whether you are Rh positive or negative
  - to test for syphilis (sexually transmitted disease)
  - to find out whether you are immune to rubella (German measles)
  - to test for sickle-cell anemia if you are of African or West-Indian descent
  - to test for thalassemia if you are of Mediterranean, African, Middle- or Far-Eastern descent

Exams:

- The doctor or midwife will feel your stomach and may do a vaginal exam (an "internal").
- The doctor may listen to your heart and lungs.

Finally:

- DON'T BE AFRAID TO ASK ANY QUESTIONS YOU WANT TO ASK
- Use this chance to put your mind at rest about anything that worries you. Get all the information you need. It can help to make a list of things you want to ask before you go for your first prenatal-care visit so nothing slips your mind.

"I was panic-stricken. It was completely unexpected. I had been told I probably wouldn't have children without some help. Just a few months before we had started thinking about whether we ought to look into in-vitro fertilization. When I told Chris, he just sat there and said, 'Well, what do we do now?'

"All our plans for the next few years were turned upside down. It took me a long time to get used to it. I walked around in shock."

This state of shock may last for a few months into the pregnancy. *"I didn't feel anything when I saw the first scan at 14 weeks. I just thought, 'Oh, yeah, a baby.' I didn't feel happy. I didn't feel anything at all."*

How a woman feels about her pregnancy—happy and confident, happy but insecure, very unhappy—may influence how soon she wants other people to know about it. Some women choose to spread the news right away, even if they had not planned to do so. *"I always thought I'd keep it quiet for the first twelve weeks. But [in fact], I wanted to tell everyone the minute I got that positive test."*

Others decide not to spread the news until the pregnancy is well established. This way, if they have a miscarriage, no one needs to be told. It's not easy to keep the secret, though. You may feel sick and almost certainly very tired. It can be hard not to explain the reason to people. *"It's tough not telling anyone for the first twelve weeks. That's when you're most vulnerable and need the most support. And that's also when you want time off work because you're so tired."*

Telling your mother can be very special. Your relationship with her will change now that you are becoming a mother yourself. As far as she is concerned, you are still her daughter. But as the mother of her grand-child, you have become something else, too. You are about to take up all the challenges and live through all the hopes and fears she herself has known. *"Rudy and I went home for Christmas. As soon as we were sitting down with my parents, I said, 'I've got something to tell you.' My mother looked at me and said, 'You're pregnant!' She was thrilled. But she did say to me later that it was funny knowing there were now two generations younger than herself."*

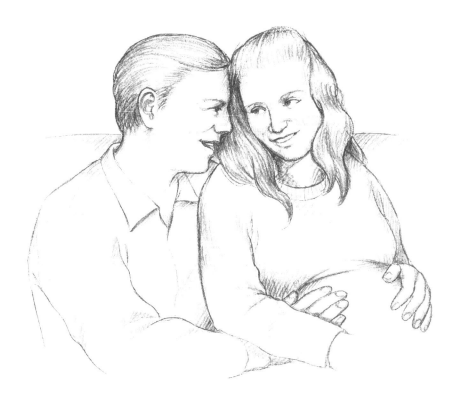

Feeling anxious during pregnancy

Even when a baby is wanted very much, pregnancy is a time when women feel many emotions. It is common to feel anxious. Women who have had problems getting pregnant may be anxious about whether they will be able to hold on to this pregnancy. Women who have had a miscarriage are often fearful until they are well beyond the latest date at which they have lost a baby. Women who have given birth to a baby who later died or who was disabled can spend an anxious nine months wondering whether the same thing might happen again. *"I was frightened all the time. I had miscarried several times. I was very worried about whether I would miscarry again. So the pregnancy caused mixed emotions in me.*

"I was most anxious in the first three months. I knew this was when most IVF ["test-tube"] babies miscarried. I was less anxious after that.

But the worry never really went away. Josh and I have the nagging guilt that we aren't meant to have a baby. We are afraid that because we've used technology to have one, we are likely to fail."

"I haven't been as happy and excited about being pregnant as I could have been. I have no idea how I'm going to cope with twins. Even though I've tried not to let the thought of what life will be like after the birth bother me, it has."

"Bella died a month after she was born with heart defects. My next pregnancy was very stressful. I had no confidence at all in having a healthy baby."

Some women really enjoy being pregnant. They sail through with no problems. Others are surprised by how strong their emotions have become. *"I can't say I have enjoyed being pregnant. I'm really looking forward to having a baby, sure. But I've been constantly aware of everything I've eaten and everything I've done for the last eight months. I've felt very aware that it's not just me I'm affecting, it's also the baby. It's a huge burden. If anything goes wrong, I'll feel like it was my fault."*

"I always used to be a calm person. That changed when I became pregnant. If I see or hear things about human suffering, or suffering involving children, I get very emotional. I cry and cry over reports of wars and famines."

Your outlook on life changes. Normal events take on a new importance. *"When I was pregnant, I remember thinking I had to be careful. If I were in an accident crossing the road, it wouldn't be just me who got hurt. In a crowd of people, I wanted plenty of space—for the two of us."*

"The bigger I get, the more aware I become. A young kid pulled out in his car right in front of me. I had to slam on the brakes to miss him. If I hadn't been pregnant, I'd have been out of the car screaming at him in no time. But I just sat still and then drove straight to my husband's work. I walked into his office and burst into tears. I was so frightened. I was thinking about our baby—not me."

Things That Might Worry You during Pregnancy

The Golden Rule Is:

If you are worried that something is wrong with your baby or you, contact your doctor or midwife or go to the hospital right away. Don't worry that there might not be a problem. It's really important that you understand what is going on and are reassured.

The problem	Questions to ask yourself so that you can inform the doctor or midwife	Possible answers What to do
Bleeding during pregnancy	When did the bleeding start? How much blood are you losing? (Do you see spots of blood? Or was there a lot of blood, like having a period?) Do you have pains in your abdomen?	Sometimes a miscarriage starts with a small amount of dark-red bleeding and stomach cramps. But during early pregnancy, it is common to have "spotting." This means you lose very small amounts of blood at the times when you normally would have had a period. Call your doctor or midwife and go to bed and rest until you can have a checkup. Is there someone you could ask to stay with you?
Sickness	Is this sickness different from morning sickness? Can you think of something you might have eaten that could have upset you? Do you feel feverish or achy? Any pains in your abdomen?	Women get minor coughs, colds and upset stomachs during pregnancy just as at any other time in their lives. But if you think your sickness may not be ordinary, see your doctor and ask for his or her advice. Be sure to see your doctor or midwife any time you feel any abdominal pain. If you don't feel well enough to go to the office or clinic, call and ask for advice. Don't give up if the clinic staff isn't very helpful. Be clear that you want to speak to or see the doctor or midwife. This is your body and your baby that you are worried about!
A fall	Did you hit your stomach or head when you fell? How do you feel now? Can you still feel the baby moving (if the fall occurred after the time you first felt your baby moving)?	A fall during pregnancy can be scary. If you're not too bruised, your head is clear and you can feel your baby moving, it's likely there's nothing to worry about. But if you are worried, or you have any pain or concussion, or your baby doesn't seem to be moving as much as he was before, call your doctor right away. And, if you can, get someone to come and look after YOU.

Things That Might Worry You during Pregnancy

Severe headaches	Do you normally get headaches? Do you see spots before your eyes? Is your vision affected by your headache? Do you feel pain in the top half of your abdomen?	Pregnancy is definitely stressful. You may get tension headaches. You may need to make time to relax, enjoy a bath, go out with your partner or friends, or treat yourself. Sometimes very bad headaches may be a symptom of a disease of pregnancy called *pregnancy-induced hypertension (PIH)* or *pre-eclampsia.* If you have spots before your eyes and pain in the upper part of your abdomen, call your doctor or midwife right away.
Baby not moving as much/not moving at all	Has today been busy and you simply have not noticed your baby moving? Have you noticed a decrease in your baby's movements over a few days? How long has it been since you last felt your baby move?	Often busy women get to the end of the day and suddenly become anxious that they haven't felt their baby move since morning. Sit or lie down and relax for an hour. See if your baby starts moving. If you are anxious at all and feel there's been a real change in the pattern of your baby's movements, call your doctor, midwife or the hospital for advice.
Waters break (the bag of waters around your baby either starts to leak or bursts with a gush of water down your legs)	If the waters broke with a gush, how much was there and at what time did they break? If the waters are trickling out, when did you first notice any wetness, or feel that you had lost some fluid other than urine into the toilet? What color is the fluid you are losing? Does it smell?	Sometimes a woman loses a small amount of water, and then the leak in the bag of waters appears to seal itself; nothing else happens. But more often, losing water from around the baby means that labor is likely to start soon and your baby is going to be born. If you are less than 37 weeks pregnant, contact the hospital right away. You will be asked to go in. If you are more than 37 weeks pregnant, you should still contact your midwife or the hospital for advice.

Pregnant women get bombarded with news from health providers and the media about what they should and should not do. They hear advice on smoking, drinking, eating, exercise, resting, taking medications. Some women can sort through the advice they get and feel confident enough to reach their own conclusions: *"I haven't worried about diet, exercise—any of it—very much. I think it's just overkill. To be honest, I've eaten blue cheese. And I understand that moderate exercise doesn't do any harm. I haven't pressured myself about that stuff."*

"It's important to be happy within yourself. You might need to make time for a leisurely walk every day with your partner or a friend. It's a good way to unwind. It lifts your spirits."

Many women become anxious and distressed. *"Pregnancy can make you feel very, very guilty. I don't drink any alcohol at all now. It's easier that way. I have friends who tell me I'm being silly, that one small glass of wine won't hurt. But this is my baby, and I'm not going to take any chances!"*

Women often need constant reassurance during their pregnancies that their babies are OK: *"At times I've felt very worried. When I was 16 weeks, I thought I should have felt the baby kick by then. So I went to see my midwife. She listened to the heartbeat and put my mind at ease. The smallest things put me into a little frenzy."*

A new self-image

Despite all the discomforts and worries of pregnancy, many women feel very positive and proud at this time. They enjoy the special attention they receive. Pregnancy says important things about you. It proclaims that you are really "grown-up." You have been sexually active and have conceived a child. You will soon be facing labor. And in a few months, you will provide 24-hour-a-day care for a new baby.

Your partner's attitude toward you may change. He may be anxious about your well-being and the well-being of his baby and show increased caution and concern. *"It was a special time. My husband didn't treat me the same. He was very caring. Not that he isn't normally caring. He was just even more so."*

Aches and Pains in Pregnancy

Pregnancy brings with it many changes in a woman's body. It is not surprising some aches and pains result. Health providers often describe these as "minor discomforts of pregnancy." They certainly do not seem minor to the woman who is suffering from them! If you have a problem during your pregnancy, ask your doctor or midwife for advice. What follows is a list of remedies women have tried over the years for pregnancy complaints and found helpful. You may not find some in textbooks. But textbooks don't always reflect the real world of women. These remedies don't work for everyone. But they're also not harmful. It may be worth a try to see if some of them work for you.

Breast Pain

One of the first signs of pregnancy is very tender breasts. Your breasts may be painful to all but the lightest touch. Try these ideas:

- Put hot or cold washcloths gently to your breasts. Putting bags of frozen peas on your breasts can also help relieve pain and tingling.
- Take plenty of hot baths or showers. Massage your breasts gently.
- Don't drink coffee, cola drinks or teas, which contain caffeine. Stay away from chocolate, too. Chocolate also contains caffeine.
- Wear a bra in bed at night. It should fit well, but not be tight. It should not have underwires.

Carpal-Tunnel Syndrome

During pregnancy, your body retains a lot of extra fluid. This is normal. But some of this fluid can cause pressure on the nerves that pass through the wrists to the hands. You may wake up in the morning with a pins-and-needles feeling in your fingers. It might be painful to hold a pen or a phone for even a short time. This problem is called *carpal-tunnel syndrome.* Most women find it goes away a few weeks after the birth of their baby.

Try these ideas:

- Swing your arms for a few minutes first thing in the morning.
- Keep your hands raised as much as you can during the day.
- Try not to write, use a keyboard or be on the phone very long.
- Soak your hands in a basin of hot or cold water.
- If you really can't stand the discomfort, ask your doctor about fitting splints for your hands and forearms.

Constipation

The hormones and pressures of pregnancy make the bowels sluggish. Constipation is common. It can cause headaches and make you feel tired. Sometimes pregnant women are prescribed iron pills because they are anemic. But too much iron can make constipation worse. So make sure you are anemic and really need to take iron pills before you start taking them. You may not need to continue taking them, either. (Research suggests that most women don't need iron tablets during pregnancy. Taking iron if you don't need it may be harmful. Yet some doctors prescribe iron pills to all their pregnant patients.) If you really do need more

continued

Aches and Pains in Pregnancy

Constipation, continued

iron, and you suffer from constipation, your doctor can prescribe a different brand. There are many.

Try the following:

- Drink lots of water.
- Eat plenty of fiber-rich foods such as whole-grain bread, cereals with bran, legumes such as lentils and beans, potatoes with their skins, brown rice.
- Eat five helpings of fruit and vegetables daily.
- Eat prunes. They are an excellent laxative.
- Don't eat eggs.
- Drink lots of pure fruit juice.
- Relax and take your time when trying to move your bowels.
- Get lots of exercise; long daily walks are excellent.

Cramps

Pregnant women often get cramps in their legs. Cramps are more likely to occur when you are in bed at night.

- Have a cup of hot or cold milk before bed. (But don't have it with chocolate!)
- Move your feet in circles and pull your toes up toward the ceiling for a few minutes before getting into bed.
- Put something under the bottom end of your mattress so that your legs are raised slightly. This will help your blood move through your feet and back up your legs during the night.
- Don't sleep flat on your back after the sixth month of pregnancy. The weight of the baby will press against a large vein (the vena cava) and slow blood circulation.

- If you get a cramp, flex your foot upwards, and massage firmly between your first and second toes. If your partner will give you a massage, that is even better!

Heartburn

Pregnancy hormones slacken the valve at the top of your stomach. This means that acid from your stomach can escape into your throat, where it causes a burning sensation. Some women find heartburn to be the worst part of pregnancy. It stops when the baby is born.

- Have small, frequent meals.
- Don't eat spicy foods or foods high in fat, such as cheese, butter, cream, fatty meat and oily fish.
- Eat a little yogurt every day. Eat some before meals, as a digestive aid.
- Drink peppermint or chamomile tea, or milk.
- Don't drink coffee or other drinks that contain caffeine, such as cola or chocolate.
- Sleep propped up on a big pile of pillows. (V-shaped pillows are great. They keep you from slipping down the bed while pregnant. And they're good for support later when you are breast-feeding your baby.)
- Try not to bend over after a meal. Squat to pick up things from the floor. You might wait to do your gardening until after your baby is born.
- Your doctor can prescribe antacids. Many women find them helpful.

continued

Aches and Pains in Pregnancy

Morning Sickness

Many women dislike the term "morning sickness" because they feel sick at all times of the day and night. It is an awful feeling. But it often goes away after about fourteen weeks of pregnancy. That's when the placenta starts making the hormones the ovaries were making until then. Some women, however, find morning sickness continues right through their pregnancies and is only cured by giving birth.

* Eat dry crackers, dry toast and anything that contains peppermint. Try nibbling on a hard gingersnap cookie.
* Have small, frequent, starchy snacks, such as bread rolls.
* Don't skip meals. Eat a little something every 2 hours, even if you don't feel like it. An empty stomach makes nausea worse. Eat a light snack, such as half a sandwich, before bed. Never skip breakfast!
* Take sips of hot water.
* Get up slowly in the morning. If possible, rest during the day.
* Stay away from smells that you know make you want to vomit.
* Wear travel-sickness bands on your wrists.
* Ask an acupuncture provider to show you the pressure point on your hand that controls nausea.

Hemorrhoids

Hemorrhoids are varicose veins in your rectum. They can make moving your bowels very painful. Lots of women find it too embarrassing to ask for help with this problem. But your doctor or midwife will be used to speaking with women about hemorrhoids. You can try the following:

* Eat a high-fiber diet rich in whole-wheat bread, legumes such as lentils and other beans, baked potatoes, fruit and vegetables.
* Don't put off going to the toilet to move your bowels. If you feel the urge to go, go!
* Drink lots of water.
* Practice your pelvic-floor exercises daily.
* Get plenty of exercise daily.
* Try an herbal hemorrhoid remedy. You can find them in a health food store (but discuss it with your doctor first).

Stretch Marks

There's no proof that any of the creams you can buy over the counter help prevent stretch marks. Stretch marks may be the way your body responds to pregnancy. But some women find that rubbing cream into their breasts, stomach and thighs makes them feel better.

If these same women don't get stretch marks, no one can say for sure if it was the cream or their bodies that did the trick! The cream will certainly soothe dry skin. If you do get stretch marks, the red lines will become pale and much less visible after your baby is born.

* Vitamin-E cream may also help after your baby is born. The oil from vitamin-E capsules, too, if applied daily, can help small scars, like stretch marks, fade.

Pelvic-Floor Exercises

These are really important! At the bottom of your pelvis is a sling of muscles that keep your bladder, uterus and rectum in the right places. This muscle helps them function well. During pregnancy, these muscles stretch because of the additional weight they support. Pregnancy hormones can also slacken them. As a result, you may find you start to wet yourself a little when you cough, sneeze or laugh. Like any other muscles in your body, your pelvic-floor muscles need to be exercised to remain strong. Women with weak pelvic-floor muscles may suffer a prolapse in their middle years. (That's when your uterus descends or "falls" into your vagina. This condition can make sexual intercourse impossible.) You can help yourself now to prevent such problems if you learn some simple exercises and practice them every day.

- Put your clenched fist to your mouth and cough into it. You should be able to feel your pelvic floor muscles bulging between your legs. These are the muscles you're going to exercise.
- Tighten the muscles around your rectum and then the muscles at the front around your vagina as if you're trying to stop yourself from passing gas (farting). Then tighten them more and more. Imagine that you have an elevator between your legs and you are taking it up to the first floor and then the second and then the third. When you are at the third floor, your muscles should be as tight as if you really needed to go to the toilet but have to wait for a while.
- Try to keep breathing while you tighten the muscles!
- Now, in stages, relax the muscles so that you come down to the second floor and then the first and then the ground floor. Don't let them crash from the third floor down to the ground!
- Try making the muscles bulge now by pushing them down to the basement. You will need to be able to do this when you are pushing your baby out into the world in the second part of labor.
- Finish the exercise by returning the muscles to their normal state on the ground floor. Repeat this exercise a few times. Tighten the muscles in stages, breathing all the time. Then let the muscles relax in stages.

To exercise all the parts that make up your pelvic-floor muscles, you also need to do the following exercise:

- Draw up your muscles as tight as you can between your legs and hold for one second; then relax. Repeat this 10 times.

Pelvic-floor muscles need daily exercise. To help yourself remember, do them each time you: have a drink, wash a dish, brush your hair, stop at traffic lights, look in a mirror, or watch an ad on TV. Do them whenever you do anything you have to do a few times a day.

The best way of testing your pelvic-floor muscles is during love-making. Your partner will be able to tell you how strong they are!

Don't test your muscles by trying to stop the flow of urine when you are on the toilet. Although women are told to do this sometimes, it may cause problems. That's because some women can't get going again after stopping the flow. But you should do your pelvic-floor muscle exercises after you've used the toilet when your bladder is empty. If you do the exercises each time you go to the bathroom, you should be doing them enough.

Eating and Drinking in Pregnancy

So much is written about what women should and should not eat during pregnancy! You may feel nervous about how to do what's best for you and your baby. It is not a good idea to "eat for two." But pregnancy can be a time when you make a special effort to enjoy a healthful, varied diet. Eat plenty of basic foods such as bread, potatoes, cereals, fruit and vegetables. In fact, you only need to avoid a few foods.

Don't eat:

- Soft cheeses such as Brie and Camembert
- Blue-veined cheeses, such as Roquefort, Gorgonzola and Stilton
- Raw and soft-boiled eggs
- Pâté and liver sausage
- Undercooked meat and poultry that is still pink
- Unwrapped foods, such as sausage rolls or tamales you are not going to heat thoroughly
- Ready-to-eat poultry
- Coleslaw and deli salads

The chances of catching listeria or salmonella from these foods are small. But there is a slight risk. And you can still eat well without having to take any risk at all.

- Liver. If you eat a lot of liver, there is a danger you will overdose on vitamin A, which could be harmful to your baby. But eating liver, including products like liverwurst, as often as once a week should not do any harm.

If you feel concerned about what you have eaten or drunk, talk to your doctor or midwife. Or call the National Center for Nutrition and Dietetics' hotline, and speak with a nutritionist. The toll-free number is: 1-800-366-1655.

Don't drink!

There is a great deal of concern about how much alcohol, if any, is safe for pregnant women to drink. Much research has shown that drinking alcohol during pregnancy can damage or kill an unborn child. Despite a great deal of study, no "safe amounts" have been determined. Therefore:

- If you are planning to conceive a baby, cut out alcohol completely.
- Don't drink any alcohol while you are pregnant. It's better to be safe than sorry.

"When I was pregnant I felt special. I was so proud, walking around with my big tummy. If we went out to the movies or to dinner, I'd stick my tummy out. I wanted the whole world to know. When I was three months pregnant, we went camping. I told everyone we met I was pregnant. I wasn't showing, but I just wanted people to know. I felt so confident. Being pregnant gave my confidence a real boost."

"I was not really happy about the weight I was putting on. But I did feel proud of myself. Pregnancy gave me a new sense of self-respect."

Exercise in Pregnancy

If you exercised before you became pregnant, there is no reason to stop now as long as both you and your baby are healthy. Sports such as sky-diving or deep-sea diving, though, are too risky during pregnancy. If either of these are your sport, it may be best to put it off until after you give birth.

Here are some guidelines about exercise in pregnancy:

- Your blood volume increases as much as 40% when you are pregnant. That means your heart has to work harder even when you are resting.

- Pregnancy is not the time to begin vigorous exercise that you have not been used to before.

- If your body tells you that you are doing too much, or you start to feel aches and pains while exercising, give yourself a break—stop for a while.

- Have plenty to drink before you start to exercise. Don't exercise in hot weather. Pregnant women need lots of fluid in their bodies. They can dehydrate easily. (This is why saunas are not good for pregnant women.)

- Sportswomen who want to train right up to the time their baby is born should check with their doctor first. Some research has shown that women who exercise at a very high level during the last weeks of pregnancy give birth to babies with low birth weights.

- A woman who is fit because exercise is a regular part of her life is likely to be well-prepared to cope with the demands of labor.

Even though they don't carry the baby themselves, partners have to live with someone who does. Men are often surprised to find how emotional the woman is during her pregnancy.

"It's hard for me to cope with her moodiness. She is grouchy and forgetful a lot of the time. And she seems to worry all *the time."*

"She's so worried about birth pain that she's gotten me really worried too."

The change in their partner's shape can also cause concern:

"I'm worried all the time about not bumping into her."

"She is really, really huge! Is that normal?"

For women, labor is a hurdle it can be hard to see beyond. But men tend to think ahead to the time after the birth. They wonder how things will change when the couple beomes a family. *"I don't know how we'll handle the changes in our lives. Our relationship will change. We'll have less money."*

Some men are anxious about their new role as father. Others are unsure about whether they really want a baby. Such men may cope during pregnancy by refusing to think about what the future holds. *"I think Roy's happy but wary. He won't think about the baby until it comes."*

Infections in Pregnancy

Once the first three months of pregnancy are over, many women feel well and remain so until the birth of their babies. Coughs and colds are always around. You don't need to worry if you catch a cold. But there are a few infections that can cause problems.

Rubella (German measles): If a woman catches rubella early in her pregnancy there is a strong chance that her baby's sight and hearing may be damaged. The later in pregnancy the virus is caught, the less dangerous it is for the baby. Your rubella immunity should be checked early in your pregnancy. Ask your doctor or midwife to tell you the result.

Varicella zoster (Chickenpox): When a woman catches chickenpox in the first half of pregnancy, her baby may be born with scars from the infection and sometimes suffers brain damage. The baby is also at risk if the mother catches chickenpox just before she is due to give birth. A pregnant mother who has chickenpox needs to see her doctor. There are treatments available that may help reduce the effect of the virus on her baby.

Toxoplasmosis: Toxoplasmosis in North America is most often caught from handling cat litter or eating undercooked meat. If the mother becomes infected during the first half of her pregnancy, her baby may be born too soon or may suffer physical damage.

You can help protect yourself from toxoplasmosis in these ways:

- Always cook meat thoroughly.
- Wash your hands after handling raw meat. Thoroughly wash any work surfaces the raw meat has touched.
- Wear gloves for gardening. Wash home-grown or store-bought vegetables before eating them.
- Wear rubber gloves to empty cat-litter trays.

Human Immunodeficiency Virus (HIV): Women who are HIV-positive run a high risk of transmitting the virus to their babies. Women with HIV need to learn about their choices in pregnancy, for birth and after their babies are born.

Sadly, fathers often have fewer chances than their partners do to talk through their feelings about pregnancy. There is little support for men who are expecting a baby, facing labor or going through early parenthood.

Feeling different and different feelings

The first three months of pregnancy are often very tiring. The baby is growing quickly, even though your stomach doesn't show yet. His world is tiny. But deep inside your pelvis, cells divide, form and move into groups. These groups become brain, heart, liver, digestive tract, kidneys, arms, legs and face in just a few days. It is no wonder that many women feel exhausted early in their pregnancy.

Morning sickness is common during these first critical months. It is worse if you skip meals or go too long without eating. (Small between-meal snacks really help!) Some women simply feel sick—not just in the morning, but at all times of the day and night. Some spend a lot of time being sick. But other women aren't bothered much by morning sickness. After all, morning sickness is just the price you sometimes have to pay for being pregnant. But it means more than that to some of us. You may find that you can no longer eat foods you once enjoyed. And you may crave things you never would have eaten before you were pregnant. Such changes in eating habits really bring home the fact that something enormous is happening to your body. *"Before getting pregnant, I had just started to try to lose weight and get fit. The healthy eating stopped when the nausea began. The thought of salads and anything green turned me off throughout my pregnancy. I felt sick for twenty weeks. But it wasn't so bad after fifteen."*

The changes pregnancy causes in your body make some women feel out of control. They have to adjust to being not quite "their own person" any more. *"I watched my body change and be examined by doctors and midwives on a regular basis. I had to cope with a new sense of myself."*

Miscarriage

Health providers call the loss of a baby before 24 weeks of pregnancy a *miscarriage*. Loss of a baby after this time is called a *stillbirth*. For the woman involved, how long she has been pregnant may not matter. *"I was thirteen weeks. They said it was an early miscarriage. It didn't feel like an early miscarriage to me."*

A miscarriage often starts with bleeding from the vagina and period-like pains. But it may be days or weeks before the woman knows she is going to lose her baby. *"When the bleeding started, I believed I knew the end result. But I had to wait a week to find out for sure on the scan. That week seemed to last forever. The scan showed the baby had died at eleven weeks. There was nothing anybody could do to console me."*

"I'd had three weeks of fluid loss and concern. I finally went in at 17 weeks with a prolapsed cord and that was it. I had the children with me. So we took them to my mom's, and my husband and I went back to the hospital. They induced me that night. I'd had three weeks of ups and downs—was it OK, or wasn't it? I guess I just wanted it to be finished."

A miscarriage that happens before 12 weeks may feel like a very unpleasant period. But if the miscarriage happens later, the woman may have to go into the hospital to give birth to her dead baby. Being in the hospital can be very upsetting. *"It's so depressing having women on the floor with you who are pregnant and just having bed rest. I cried and cried when I heard them listening to the baby's heartbeat in the next bed."*

Some women choose to go home first. It can help to spend a few days getting ready before coming into the hospital for the labor. *"When we went for my scan, he was dead and we didn't know. I mean he kicked that morning and I went for my 20-week scan and he was dead. They*

Miscarriage
(Losing a baby before 24 weeks of pregnancy)

What to look for:

• *Bleeding from the vagina*—brownish spots or bright-red bleeding

• *Pain*—period-like pains that come and go

• *Backache*—felt low in the back

What to do:

• Contact your doctor or midwife and ask for advice.

• Rest in bed or stay up, but take it easy. (It has not been proved that lying in bed helps prevent a miscarriage. This advice is often given, though, and may make you feel better.)

• Don't have intercourse if you are bleeding or spotting.

• Ask your partner, a good friend or your mother to be with you.

What will happen:

• You have to wait and see. That is the hardest part of all.

• If you keep bleeding and the flow gets heavier, a miscarriage is likely.

• If you have a lot of severe pain and very heavy bleeding, you may be taken to the hospital until the miscarriage happens.

• The bleeding may lessen and the pregnancy could continue normally.

Taking care of *you*

Whether you lose the baby or the pregnancy settles down again, you will have had a great shock. You will need and deserve lots of support:

• Find a friend you can talk to about what's happened. (Your partner may be as shocked as you are and not able to support you at this time.)

• Ask your doctor or midwife to explain anything you don't understand.

• Contact Sidelines, a nonprofit agency for women having a problem pregnancy. Call Tracy Hoogenbloom at (909) 563-6199, or Candace Hurley at (714) 497-2265. Ask to be put in touch with someone who has been through the same thing who can support you.

said, *'We can induce labor now or you can go home and prepare your-self. We suggest you go home.' That was what I wanted, too. I needed time to think about what had happened and what would happen."*

Telling other people about a miscarriage adds to the trauma. It can be hard when children need to be told: *"Telling our daughter was tough. She was looking forward to the new baby so much."*

But children often accept such events better than adults. Adults may find it hard to respond to such distressing news: *"Maybe they didn't want to upset me, but they made* no comment at all *about the miscarriage. And later, when I met them in the street, they just gave me a quick glance. I felt like I had done something wrong and it was all my fault."*

Parents who have miscarried their baby need to have their loss acknowledged: *"A few words would have been much better than none."*

The Second Half of Pregnancy

In the second half of pregnancy, as your tummy gets bigger, problems may begin that relate to your increasing weight. Your legs may ache or cramp. Varicose veins and hemorrhoids may appear. The hormones of pregnancy slacken the valve at the top of the stomach. Acid from the stomach may back up into your throat and cause heartburn. Eating yogurt once or twice a day often relieves heartburn in pregnancy. Most women, if they have people to support them, cope well with these discomforts. But the discomforts can still be very unpleasant. *"The constipation that was an ongoing feature of my pregnancy got worse. I started to have difficulty with hemorrhoids. The fiber supplement from the doctor just about got me going, but not quite. Because I hadn't wanted to eat vegetables since I became pregnant, and drinking fruit juice gave me heartburn, there wasn't much I could do to help myself. I had to grin and bear it."*

Women like to take care of themselves while they are pregnant. It is a time when many reassess their lives and try to become more health-conscious. Things that might have been too much trouble to do when you were not pregnant, such as giving up smoking or starting to exercise, often become possible at this time. You know your baby will benefit from a healthful lifestyle. Better eating habits, getting more rest and making an effort to swim or walk a couple of times a week can make you feel better, too.

"I felt healthier every day. I ate decent food and read and relaxed."

"The swimming toned my body. I had no problems carrying my ever-growing tummy."

The middle part of a first pregnancy may be one of the most pleasant times of a woman's life. Labor still seems too far in the future to worry about. There is the excitement of feeling the baby moving. And later on, the baby will be kicking day and night!

"I loved my growing tummy. I spent hours stroking it and wondering what the baby would be like."

Toward the end of pregnancy, the tiredness that was a feature of the first few weeks comes back. Being pregnant and still having to go to work can be exhausting. Many women long for the day when their maternity leave will begin. *"I couldn't cope with the trip to work by train any longer—I had to make three transfers. Instead, I left home in the car at 7 a.m. to miss the traffic. I'd swim at the workout center near the office. Then I'd get to the office in time to eat breakfast before starting work."*

During the last three months of pregnancy, some women take over all the pillows in the house at night. They might put one under their tummy, one between their legs, one in the small of their back and a couple of others under their head. It may seem hard to get comfortable enough to get to sleep. Turning over in bed becomes a big problem. Partners often decide they have a better chance of getting a good night's sleep if they move to a sofa or a spare room for a while!

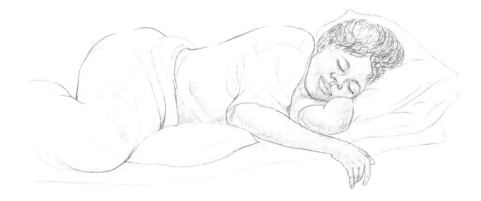

Your Baby's Growth and Development

First Three Months of Pregnancy

- Your baby grows very quickly.
- His heart begins to beat.
- His blood circulates through his body.
- He can suck, swallow and urinate.
- His arms and legs start to form.
- His face starts to develop.
- He starts to move.

Second Three Months of Pregnancy

- You start to feel your baby's first movements. As he grows, his movements become more vigorous.
- Your baby's heart can be heard with a stethoscope through the wall of your tummy. (You can hear it, too, if you ask to use the stethoscope.)
- The two sections that form the hard palate inside your baby's mouth connect.

- Your baby's fingernails start to grow.
- He develops his own pattern of sleeping and waking. You will learn when he is active and when he is resting.
- He can hear and will "jump" if there is a sudden loud noise.
- His eyes are open.

Last Three Months of Pregnancy

- Your baby starts to make breathing movements.
- His skin becomes smoother—less wrinkled and hairy.
- His nails and hair grow longer and his skull hardens.
- His body becomes rounder and plumper as he puts down fat stores to prepare for labor and the first few days of his life.

The Nine-Month Miracle

The First Trimester

Your baby may seem to grow up very quickly after he is born, but never again will he grow and change as quickly as he did in your womb. When you have been pregnant for three weeks, your baby is about the size of a pea. He's just a cluster of cells. But those cells contain the amazing potential to become the fully formed person who will be your unique child. By the time you are 12 weeks pregnant—before you start to show!—your baby is the size of an avocado. But his heart, blood vessels, kidneys, gut, sex organs, nervous system, head and face, arms and legs are all formed. His heart is beating. His blood is flowing through his body. He can suck, swallow and pee.

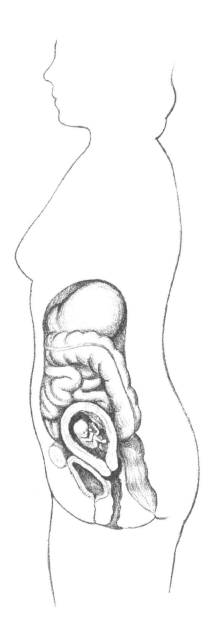

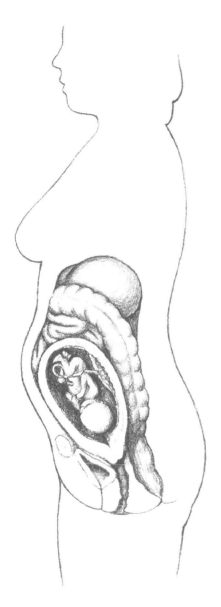

The Second Trimester

During the rest of your pregnancy, your baby will simply grow in size and practice using his body. You will be able to feel him moving from the time you are about 18 to 22 weeks pregnant if this is your first pregnancy. You may feel movement sooner if this is your second pregnancy. But actually, your baby has been moving since he was two months old. By five months of pregnancy, your baby can hear your voice. Talk to him! By 6-1/2 months, his eyes are open. As your tummy stretches, he can tell light from dark.

The Third Trimester

During his last three months in the womb, your baby's nails will grow to the end of his fingertips—and beyond. His hair gets longer, too. He becomes much fatter to prepare for the hard work of being born and for life in the outside world.

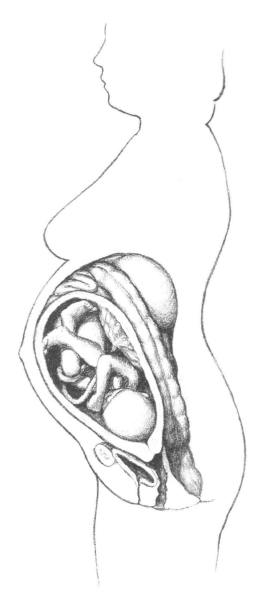

Drugs in Pregnancy

Street Drugs

Much of the research about what happens to babies when their mothers use street drugs during pregnancy has involved small numbers of women and their babies. There is equally little research on women who often use street drugs compared with those who sometimes use them. Our knowledge of street drugs and pregnancy is limited in some important ways. But there is little doubt street drugs cause many problems for babies. No one is likely to care more about an unborn child than the woman who is carrying him. If a pregnant woman is using an illegal drug, the best thing she can do for her baby is get help. A healthcare professional can provide referrals for help and counseling.

What follows is a list of some of the risks to babies if their mothers take illegal drugs.

Amphetamines and Ecstasy

Babies are at risk of:
• Being born too early
• Being born very small
• Having a cleft palate
• Having heart problems
• Having a mental disorder

Cannabis (Marijuana, Pot)

Babies are at risk of:
• Being born too early
• Being born too small
• Being very jumpy and hard to settle in the first weeks of their lives
• Slow development in the first years of life

Cocaine

Babies are at risk of:
• Dying in the womb because their mothers develop serious blood-pressure problems
• Being born with gangrenous (seriously infected) toes and fingers
• Having heart and kidney problems
• Being extremely fussy in the first weeks of life. Such babies often require special care to help them cope with withdrawal symptoms.

We do know that even women who are not addicted to cocaine and use it only now and then put their babies at serious risk.

Heroin

Babies are at risk of:
• Being born too early
• Being very small and sickly
• Needing treatment to help them cope with withdrawal symptoms
• Slow physical and mental development in the first years of life

LSD

It's still not certain what effect LSD has on unborn and newborn babies. There don't seem to be more problems among babies born to women who use LSD. But other substances are often mixed with illegal LSD. These may be harmful to babies.

Solvents and Glue

Babies are at risk of:
• Being very small and short at birth
• Having kidney and bladder problems

Methadone

Methadone can be legally obtained by heroin addicts and addicts of other drugs. It carries its own risks. Women who use methadone are more likely to miscarry. If their babies survive, they tend to be slow to develop in the first years of life. They do seem to catch up with other "normal" children by the time they are two or three years old.

Drugs in Pregnancy

Over-the-Counter (OTC) Drugs

Many people take drugs on a daily basis. Drugs such as aspirin and acetaminophen (Tylenol®), cough syrups and cold remedies, laxatives and caffeine, are widely used. People who use these drugs may not think they are using drugs, but they are!

A quick look in the medicine cabinet at home is likely to reveal lots of tablets and mixtures such as cough syrup. Many of them may be out of date. You may have bottles with no labels on them, and you can't quite remember what they contain. Pregnancy is a good time to go through your medicine cabinet. Throw out anything in it you are uncertain about.

A few over-the-counter or prescription drugs are known to be harmful to unborn babies. (Some of these are drugs women have to take when they are pregnant, such as drugs for epilepsy.) But it is wise to be especially cautious about what you take during pregnancy. Ask your doctor or local pharmacist about any tablet or medicine you are thinking of taking. (Pharmacists can provide excellent, up-to-date information on drugs.)

Cut down on drinks containing caffeine (mainly coffee and cola). And be careful until your baby is born. If you breast-feed, continue to be careful until your baby is no longer feeding from you.

Whatever drugs you take, your unborn or breast-feeding baby will be taking them, too.

Waiting for Labor to Start

Pregnancy is full of dreams about what the baby will be like. Most people experience a lot of worry about whether the baby will be healthy. Fears of having a baby who is not normal or who is born dead can cause a lot of distress. *"I have this recurring nightmare: I'm giving birth and the baby gets stuck inside me. The doctor yanks him out and he's dead."*

"I'm going to accept whatever comes along in labor as long as the baby and I are OK. Of course, I have an ideal birth in my mind and an ideal baby. Hopefully they will happen."

Some women don't let themselves think too much about labor in case the baby is not born healthy: *"I don't think about the birth in case something goes wrong. It's a defense I have put up."*

Other women always seem to be serene and confident: *"I have never wondered whether the baby will be OK. I just know he will. I often put headphones on my stomach and play the baby music. I tell him about the things we'll do together."*

Smoking in Pregnancy

Mothers who smoke during pregnancy and after their babies are born are not doing themselves or their babies any good. Smoking cuts the supply of oxygen available to the baby while he is in the uterus.

Babies are more likely to die in the womb or at birth if their mothers smoke. They can also be born too soon and are sometimes small and sickly. After birth, these babies are at greater risk of sudden infant death (SIDS) because they live in a smoky environment.

Sometimes it's too hard for women to give up smoking, even though they want to do what is right for their babies. So:

• If you can give up, do.

• If you think you could give up, get all the help you can from your doctor or midwife, and from your partner and friends.

• If you can't give up, try to cut down. Each cigarette you *don't* smoke is going to be better for your baby.

It can be hard to imagine what you will feel like when your baby is born and first put into your arms. During pregnancy, the baby has a fantasy life. That means she can be whatever her mother wants her to be. As the moment of birth nears, women have to replace the fantasy with reality.

"I try not to think about how I'll feel when I meet my baby. I might be disappointed. I'll just wait and see what happens at the time and not expect too much. It could be one extreme or the other."

"I really love my baby already. Whether I'll feel like that when it's born, I'm not sure."

Some people would strongly prefer to have a baby of one sex or the other. The end of pregnancy is the time when you have to accept the fact that such a dream may not come true. *"Every time I've dreamed about the baby, it's been a boy. I think it has something to do with the fact we'd both like a girl. I think it's my way of trying to come to terms with the fact that it might be a boy."*

Once labor is only a few weeks away, women start to face up to the business of giving birth. It is likely they will have heard a lot of stories about labor. They may have been very frightened by some of them. Women can be unkind to other women who have not yet had babies. They often describe (or exaggerate) their labors. But it is likely that women at all times and in all cultures have looked forward to labor with a mixture of eagerness and dread.

"You don't know what you are going to feel."

"*I'm trying to be positive. I don't really know what it is going to feel like. I think it might be like going for a long walk up a mountain when you don't know if you're getting near the top.*"

"*I'm not looking forward to the labor and birth. I'm worried about how painful it's going to be. I'm looking forward to after the birth when I've got the baby.*"

"*It can't be that bad or the population of the planet would be dwindling.*"

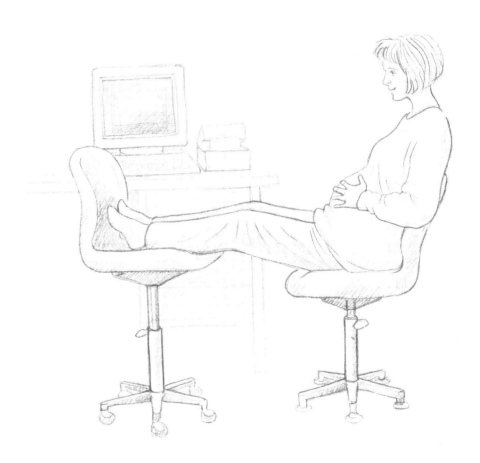

If the day on which the baby is due arrives and passes without labor starting, women may find themselves the objects of unwanted attention. Friends and relatives start calling to ask whether the baby has come yet. The last few weeks can seem very long. Women often become anxious for labor to start. *"It somehow seems better if it comes early. Waiting for labor, when it's late, is dreadful. You feel so big and you can't sleep. There's the excitement of it. You think you might be having contractions. Then they go away and you realize that it wasn't IT."*

"I really enjoyed the last few weeks of my pregnancy, puttering around. My due date came and so did my mother, who was going to help us after the birth. But the baby didn't come. Each day, Michael and Mom would empty and refill the birthing pool and get things ready to go. I felt as if I were in limbo. I didn't really believe I was going to meet the baby inside me."

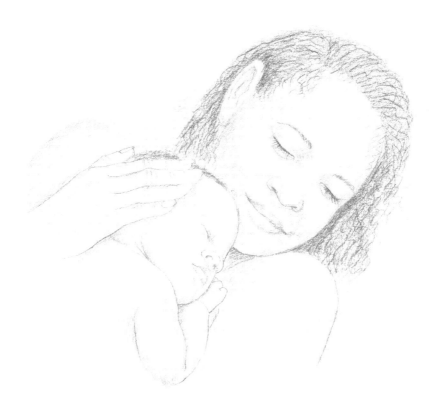

Many women—and more men!—are frightened that they will not know when labor has started. Talk to other parents and to midwives and health providers. Read books and go to childbirth classes. Then you'll learn what to expect. You may still have false alarms and think you are in labor when you are not. But the day will come when you will be quite sure. *"People used to say I'd know when labor had started. I didn't believe them. But they were right—I did!"*

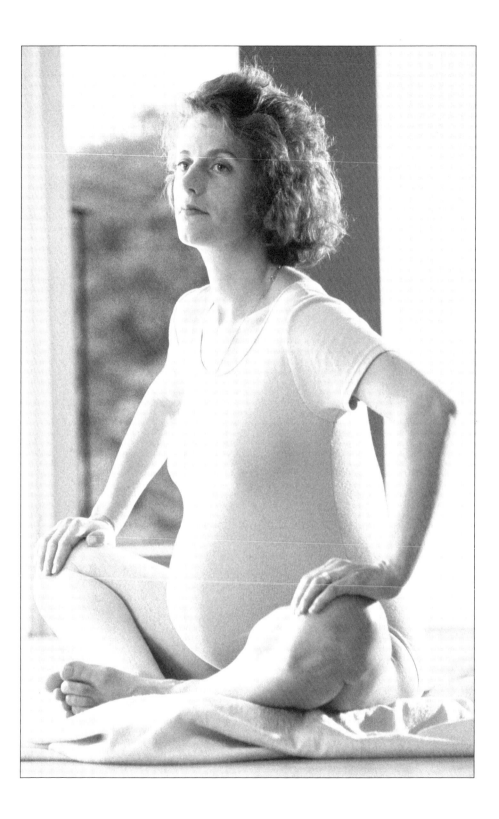

CHAPTER 2 *Choosing Where Your Baby Will Be Born*

How do people make choices about health care? How does a pregnant woman decide whether her baby should be born at home, in a birth center or in a hospital? There are all sorts of pressures at work upon her. She will be aware of some of them. But some will affect her unconsciously. She may be influenced by what she has seen on TV and in the movies. She may be affected by newspaper articles, magazines and books she has read. Perhaps most of all, she may be influenced by her own mother and where she had her babies. If her mother had home births and enjoyed them, or had hospital births and felt good about them, she may believe she will be happy with the same thing:

"I think because my mother had all of us at home, a home birth sounded right for me."

"I was born in a hospital, even though it was less common then. My mother had no problems at all."

A woman may be influenced by her sister(s) or other relatives. The stories she is told by her close friends about the local hospitals or birth centers may make a difference to her: *"My friend gave birth at a birth center. She had a very positive birth. I'm sure that influenced me."*

"My sisters had their babies in a hospital. It seemed to me they had one intervention after another. That soured me on having my baby in a hospital."

"I went to the local hospital because my two closest girlfriends had their babies there. It was a wonderful hospital."

Most women choose to give birth in a hospital because they think a hospital is the safest place for a baby to be born. Women in other countries don't feel the same way. In Holland, for instance, it is still common to give birth at home. The government provides women with home nurses for a few weeks after they have given birth. Recent studies in the United States and England have shown that home birth is as safe as hospital births for healthy mothers with normal pregnancies. In fact, studies show that infants born at home do better (have higher Apgar scores) than those born in hospitals. Mothers who give birth at home have fewer vaginal tears and fewer medical interventions. There is no clear evidence that having babies away from hospitals is less safe for women with normal pregnancies. It may be that mothers (and doctors) will begin to rethink their attitude towards home birth. More women will choose this option when more doctors and midwives decide to attend births in the home. But in some parts of the United States few healthcare providers attend home births. Often, the reason is that they cannot get insurance to cover a home-birth practice.

Getting Informed and Becoming Confident

Women who want to make choices about the kind of care they receive in pregnancy and during labor may have to do their own research. At first you may not know exactly what you want. You may not know what your options are. You may never have been in a hospital in your life. You may never have had any medical tests. You may never have spoken to a midwife or held a newborn baby. But you will soon become very much more aware! Once you are pregnant, you start to notice things on TV and in the papers about birth and babies. You also start to speak with friends who have had babies. You go to clinics where you talk to other pregnant women about the choices they have made. And you attend prenatal classes where you can gain a lot of knowledge.

"This is my first pregnancy. There's a lot I don't know. It has really helped to go to the classes. I've had a chance to talk through all the choices and options with other women and the teacher. This has really helped me think about the kind of birth I want."

Your Choices for Pregnancy and Birth

Ask yourself:

• *Would you prefer to receive most of your pre- and postpartum care from your family doctor?* Your family doctor may also be able to attend your birth, at home or in the hospital. If not, your family doctor may refer you to an obstetrician or a midwife with whom he or she is used to working.

• *Would you rather give birth in a birth center than at home or in a hospital?* Birth centers can be freestanding or part of a larger hospital. They are designed for women with normal pregnancies and births. Birth centers offer a limited number of interventions. They are set up to provide the comforts of home, such as showers or baths, and a private room. If you sign up for a birth-center birth, you may have to attend prenatal classes. Such classes are often given at the birth center itself. But they may also be given by private teachers.

• *Would you prefer to see an obstetrician for your care?* Obstetricians often work in groups. You will see one or another of them when you come into the office for prenatal care. By the time you are ready to give birth, you probably will have met them all. Then, when you are in labor, the doctor in the group whose turn it is to be on call will attend you.

HMOs have an increasing number of programs. Some provide for each mother to be cared for by just one doctor or midwife. Ask if such a program is provided through your health plan.

• *Would you prefer to receive most of your pre- and postpartum care from a small team of midwives whom you can get to know?* One of them will help you give birth. (Many HMOs are starting to organize nurse-midwives into teams. This may be an option for you.)

• *Would you like to have a certified nurse-midwife care for you?* You may be able to see the same midwife throughout your pregnancy, in labor and until a few weeks after your baby is born. You may be able to give birth at home, in a birth center or in a hospital. The nurse-midwife will explain the choices available in your area. Your nurse-midwife is likely to arrange back-up care with an obstetrician in case problems come up during pregnancy or labor. But she (or he) is fully qualified to care for you throughout a normal pregnancy and birth.

You will be swamped with information. Soon you will be able to decide for yourself about things such as where to have your baby. If, in the middle or even at the end of your pregnancy, you want to change your mind, there is no reason why you can't: *"When we went to sign up at the Health Center, the doctor said to me: 'You're over thirty, so you won't want to have your baby at home. Your options are to go to hospital a, b or c.' I said, 'OK, that's fine.' Later on, I got worried because I don't like hospitals. Someone mentioned home birth so I started finding out about it. I went to a home birth support-group meeting. Suddenly it all felt right and I decided to go for it."*

Making Tough Choices

When it comes to making choices, you have to feel confident that you know what is right for you: *"To get the choices you want, you don't ask, you just say. But you have to feel confident."*

Feeling confident is hard if you've given birth with difficulty before. In such cases, women often choose to have a different type of care from what they might once have preferred: *"I wanted a home birth with my first pregnancy. I was amazed at the opposition I had. But then I had a late miscarriage and we moved to a new area. Home didn't really feel like home. I panicked when I became pregnant again. My feelings changed completely. I thought, 'I don't care where this baby is born as long as it's born alive.' When I met my doctor for the first time, she assumed I'd want all the technology there was. Home birth wasn't even discussed. I just signed up at the hospital and she kept a really close eye on me. I was pleased with that."*

"I had all kinds of interventions during my first labor. One just led to another and then another. I'm very anxious not to do the same this time. I'd like to have a home birth and not go near a hospital. But, because I had all those interventions the first time around, part of me wouldn't like to risk a home birth. So I've chosen to give birth in a birth center."

In cases like these, decisions depend on weighing what you would most like against what will make you feel most secure. As long as the final choice is yours, you are likely to feel better about it than if someone else chooses for you.

Choosing a home birth

Women who choose to have a home birth give all sorts of reasons. Some simply know in their heart that this is where their baby should be born. Others feel that they will be more relaxed in their own home. Some cherish the privacy they can have at home and the freedom to do as they choose. Some worry about their baby being exposed to dangerous germs in hospitals, because hospitals take care of very sick people. Some find hospitals frightening. They fear they are more likely to have a lot of interventions if they have their babies there:

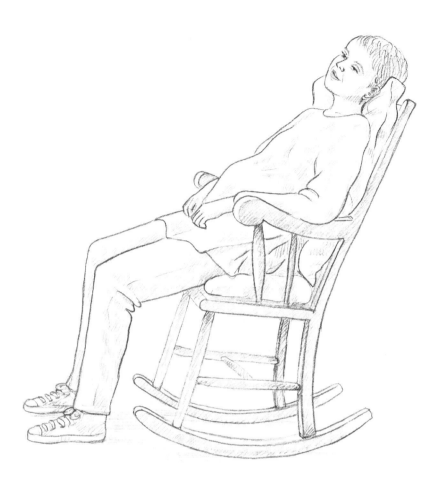

"I've chosen a home birth. I want as few interventions as possible. I'd like help—a LOT of help—but as few interventions as possible."

"One of the main reasons I wanted to have my baby at home is that I felt if I went into the hospital with strangers around, I wouldn't be very assertive. I thought if the midwife came to my house, she'd be much more likely to ask me before doing something."

"The thing about home birth is working one-on-one with the midwife. The midwife who comes to my home will be with me throughout the length of my labor."

"I can have candlelight if I want to. I can wander around the house and make as much noise as I want! Whatever I need is here."

"I just knew I wanted my babies at home."

Where Do You Want Your Baby to Be Born?

This is an important decision, which you will be asked to make at the start of your pregnancy. You can always change your mind later if you want to. Keep in mind:

Home Birth

- Will you be more relaxed in labor if you are in your own home where you can do what you please?

- Would you prefer the doctor or midwife to be a guest in your house rather than you being a "guest" at the hospital?

- Will you feel safer at home?

- Do you want to have as little medical intervention during your labor as possible?

- How does your partner feel about home birth?

- Is your home a good place to give birth? (Is there a phone? Is there a place where you can be quiet? Is there heating in the room where the baby will be born? Is there a private bathroom and hot water? Can you make plans for your other children to be cared for elsewhere if you don't want them to be with you at the birth?)

- Can you afford the cost of a home birth? If you have health insurance, will your insurance plan cover the fee of your home-birth doctor or midwife?

Birth-Center Birth

- Would you feel more secure giving birth in a birth center?

- Birth centers provide many of the comforts of home plus the safety of medical technology.

- Do you want your older children or other family members or friends present at your birth? Birth centers are often more flexible than hospitals about the number of people who may attend a birth, and their ages.

- Does your HMO operate a birth center? Will your health insurance cover the costs of a birth-center birth?

- Do you want to have a great deal of control about how your labor is managed? If your home does not seem right for a home birth, but you want the freedom to move about and manage your labor in your own way, then a birth center may be the best choice for you.

Hospital Birth

- Will you be more relaxed in labor if you are in a hospital where there are always doctors and midwives around?

- Will you feel safer in a hospital?

- How does your partner feel about hospital birth?

- Will the hospital help you have the kind of birth you want to have?

If you choose to have your baby in a hospital, you might want to think about which hospital to use. There may be more than one in your area.

Ask yourself:

- What have you heard about the local hospitals from other women who have recently given birth? This kind of knowledge can be very helpful. Women who have given birth at a certain hospital really know what it is like!

- Is one hospital or one doctor known for using a lot of medical procedures during labor? Are there others who are known for letting women do what they want?

continued

Where Do You Want Your Baby to Be Born?

Hospital Birth, continued

- Which attitude would suit you better? You should be able to get statistics about such things as how many women have:

  – their labors induced

  – Cesarean sections

  – forceps deliveries

  – episiotomies (snipping a woman's vaginal opening with scissors to widen it)

You should be able to find out these things from the hospitals themselves.

You can also find out about the intervention rates of particular doctors. Ask at the hospital where she delivers babies. Or ask the doctor herself.

You might want to think about these things when choosing among hospitals and doctors:

- How easy is it for you to get to each of the local hospitals?

- Is there one that seems better maintained, more up to date and nicer?

- Are some hospitals eager to send women home quickly after their babies are born just because they have too few beds?

- Do any of the local hospitals have a birthing pool so that you can use a warm bath to help you cope with pain in labor?

"I wasn't really sure why I wanted to have my baby at home. But I could see 110 reasons not to go into the hospital. I used to get annoyed when people asked, 'Why are you having it at home?' I'd just say, 'Why not?'"

If your partner or someone else is going to support you during labor, they need to be happy with your choice of a home birth, too. Someone who is frightened of the place in which you have chosen to labor may not be able to give you the support you need. They may feel the place you have chosen is too clinical, or not clinical enough. Talk through where you want your baby to be born. Allow the labor-support person you choose to gather his own data. This often results in a choice you can both accept: *"My partner wasn't eager to try a home birth. I explained my thinking to him and let him talk to other people about home births. I didn't push him. I didn't want him to be unhappy. He was going to be a very important person to me in labor. In the end, he came around by listening to other people who'd had their babies at home."*

Choosing to have a home birth can sometimes be made harder because of resistance from healthcare providers: *"I was surprised by my doctor's negative attitude. He discussed the three local hospitals with me. But he stated firmly that he would not be happy for me to have a home birth."*

Although attitudes towards home birth are changing among healthcare providers, some doctors and nurses still prefer not to care for a woman who wants to have her baby at home. After all, healthcare providers do most of their training in hospitals. And in some places, doctors and midwives cannot obtain insurance if they attend home births. Your doctor may explain to you that he cannot care for you if you want a home birth. But he may be happy to refer you to a doctor or midwife who can: *"My doctor said he was happy to care for me during my pregnancy and after the birth. He said he'd find another doctor from the practice who would cover me for a home birth."*

"I'm lucky enough to live in a place where it is fairly easy to find a home-birth provider. Although my doctor chose not to be involved, he didn't try to talk me out of it. I had my prenatal care with a midwife. I was very happy with it. My midwife agreed to a home birth even though they had used forceps with my first child. She was extremely positive about the whole thing."

Choosing a hospital birth

Women who choose to have their babies in a hospital feel more secure knowing there will be lots of doctors and nurses around. Some feel that using medical technology is likely to make a birth safer:

"I chose a hospital because it was my first child. I'm not very brave, and I wanted as many people there as possible to help me."

"I wouldn't feel relaxed having a baby at home even if I knew I was having a full-term, healthy baby. I would like to be in a hospital with all the doctors, nurses and equipment."

"I decided early on that I wanted a hospital birth instead of a home birth. We wanted to reduce the risk. We made a joint decision. I didn't go to look at any of the hospitals. I just went for the one that was nearest."

"I decided to go to the nearest hospital. Once you've seen the people there a few times, they seem human enough. That makes all the difference. I made the decision on gut reactions."

"I feel that things are suggested at the hospital, but are in no way forced on you. I'm happy with that."

If you are thinking about giving birth in a hospital, both you and the person who will provide your labor support should be happy about the choice: *"I wanted to go to the hospital in case something went wrong. My husband thought that would be best, too."*

Choosing a Birth-Center Birth

Women who choose to give birth in a birth center seek the comforts of a home-like setting. Birth centers provide women the freedom to choose for themselves how their labors and births will be managed. They also feel more secure knowing the birth center is equipped to respond to emergencies. Some birth centers are set up just for births. Others are sites at which women may also receive prenatal care.

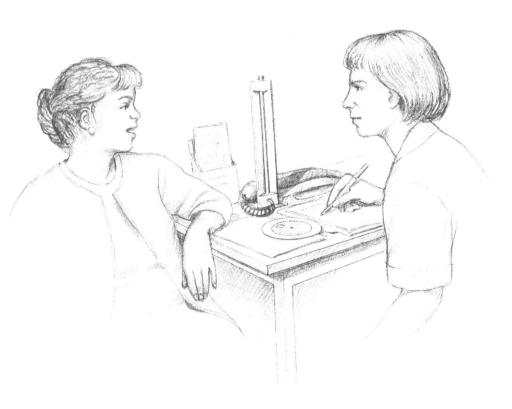

Changing Childbirth: The View from Great Britain

In 1991, the British government set up a task force to review maternity services in England. The committee heard the views of midwives, obstetricians, pediatricians, health and social-service personnel, dietitians and nurses. The committee also listened to many women who spoke about their own pregnancies and births. Groups involved in issues surrounding pregnancy and birth spoke at length to the committee about the kind of care they felt women wanted.

A summary of the committee's findings was published in 1992. It stressed that healthcare providers should not presume to know what is best for any single woman. Instead, they should provide information to help women make their own choices about the kind of care they want. The committee felt that midwives should care for women who have normal pregnancies and births. Obstetricians should only care for the few women who have complicated pregnancies.

The committee decided there was no evidence to suggest that home birth is unsafe for healthy women. Healthcare providers were asked to ensure that each woman knows she has the right to choose to have her baby at home.

Based on the committee's report, known as the *Winterton Report,* the British government set up an Expert Maternity Group to consider the report's findings. This group published its own report in 1993 called *Changing Childbirth.*

Changing Childbirth states that:

"The woman must be the focus of maternity care. She should be able to feel that she is in control of what is happening to her and able to make decisions about her care, based on her needs, having discussed matters fully with the professionals involved."

The essence of *Changing Childbirth* is captured in the three "Cs"—Choice, Control and Continuity:

CHOICE: A woman should be able to choose the type of care that she feels is best for her. She could choose to give birth at home, in a birth center or in a hospital. She could choose to receive her care from a doctor or a midwife.

CONTROL: She should feel in control of what happens to her. That's because she helps make the decisions about her care.

CONTINUITY: She should be able to get to know a small group of healthcare providers during her pregnancy. The same people should care for her until a few weeks after her baby is born. Childbearing women shouldn't have to meet a new provider at each stage of their care.

Changing Childbirth is an exciting document. In Britain, it has become a Bill of Rights for childbearing women. Maternity services are now being planned to comply with its views. And British women should soon be able to have more say in their care than they have ever had before.

If you want to give birth in a birth center, you may have to search a little to locate one. Even after you find one, you may have to be persistent in order to get signed up to give birth there.

"When I first went to the doctor and said I wanted to give birth in the birth center, he wrote on my chart that he didn't think I was suitable. But when I saw the midwife, she said, 'Of course you can, no problem.'"

"I went to my first prenatal visit and I asked about a birth-center birth. The midwife said it was not a good idea because I was having my first baby. I'd be tired after the birth, and it would be much better if I stayed in the hospital. But I stuck to my guns. I'm glad I did. I feel that a hospital isn't a very good place to recover. I recovered much better in the birth center and at home."

"That's the good thing about the birth center: You go in with the midwife when she thinks you're ready and then you leave within six hours after the birth. So you use the birth center, have your own midwife, and get home quickly—ideal. And it costs less, too!"

Current research suggests that women should see just a few doctors or midwives for their maternity care. With some health plans you may see a new doctor or midwife at each prenatal visit. Then another doctor or midwife may help you give birth. This makes it hard for the healthcare providers to get to know you and for you to get to know them.

If you are paying the bills yourself or if you have health insurance that permits you to shop around, by all means do so! Look for a small team of doctors or midwives who will take care of you from the time you find out you are pregnant until after the birth of your baby. This will make it much easier for you to learn about your choices for birth, to ask questions and to feel relaxed with your caregivers.

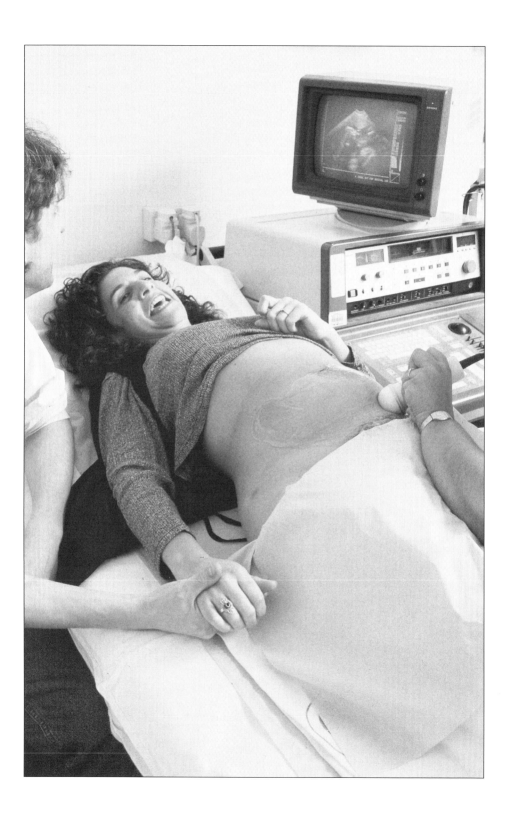

CHAPTER 3 *Prenatal Testing*

Expecting a baby may have been easier for our mothers and grand-mothers than it is for women today. Our mothers were often not certain they were pregnant until they had missed at least a few periods. Today, it is possible to know within days of having sex whether or not you have become pregnant. This means that during the first three months of pregnancy, when it is common to miscarry, women are now fully aware that they are losing a baby. It used to be that they would either never have known they were pregnant, or they would not have been sure.

Most women today do not imagine that their babies might die. A hundred years ago women knew that this was very possible. Women now choose, for the most part, to have only one or two pregnancies. And many choose not to start a family until they are in their late twenties, their thirties or even forties. So it is really important that their few babies are healthy. To help ensure that women bear healthy infants, a whole range of prenatal tests have been developed. They try to detect whether an unborn baby has a problem, such as spina bifida or Down syndrome, which can affect him after birth.

These tests carry with them all sorts of choices for the woman and her partner. The hardest choice of all can be whether or not to end a pregnancy. But there are other tough decisions to make, too. You may have to decide which test carries the least risk for the mother and her baby. You may have to learn at what stage in pregnancy it is best to have tests. And you may have to decide whether to have a second test to confirm the results of a first test.

To make such choices, you have to understand the concept of risk. But that's not so easy to do. Screening tests do not tell you whether your baby has a certain condition for sure. They only show how likely he is to have that condition. The mother who looks at a test report which states that her risk of carrying a baby with Down syndrome is 1 in 180 may find this result hard to grasp. One in 180 doesn't sound very high. But because it is a greater risk than the test's cut-off point of 1 in 250, she has been told that her blood test is "positive." That makes it sound as though the risk is very great indeed. She may ask herself what it might mean to her to have a baby with Down syndrome or what it might mean to her to end her pregnancy.

The choices that need to be made about prenatal testing are not small. They may well affect you, in one way or another, for the rest of your life. It is vital that you get support while you are making choices about testing. You can speak with your doctor, midwife, partner, friends and other women who have been through the same tests. Learn as much as you can. Many women don't ask questions. Then they look back and wonder why they made the choices they did.

Getting Informed

How much a pregnant woman learns about the different tests she can have can vary. Sometimes you may only find out about a kind of test by chance: *"I picked up a magazine and read about CVS (chorionic villus sampling). I thought, 'Gosh, that sounds better than amniocentesis because it's so much earlier.' I asked to have it, but it was never suggested to me."*

Prenatal Testing: Screening or Diagnostic

It's important to understand the difference between a SCREENING test and a DIAGNOSTIC test:

A **screening test** tells you whether you are at increased *risk* of having a baby with a certain condition, such as Down syndrome. It does not tell you whether your baby has Down syndrome (or any other condition). To know for sure, you need to have a diagnostic test.

A **diagnostic test** tells you for sure whether your baby has certain conditions, such as Down syndrome or spina bifida.

Other women find that healthcare providers spend a lot of time talking to them about tests: *"At my first prenatal visit, the midwife talked with me in some detail about my options for testing. She also went over what we could do afterward, depending on the results. My family doctor also talked about tests with me."*

"I asked my doctor to refer me for a CVS test, which she did. A few days later, a midwife called from the hospital. We had a very long talk. We discussed the risk of losing the baby because of the tests. We also talked about the risk of my carrying a baby with Down syndrome based on my

Some Conditions Prenatal Tests Can Detect

These are some of the more common conditions that prenatal tests can detect. Other rare conditions can be picked up as well.

Down syndrome

This is a condition caused by an "abnormal chromosome." This means something is wrong with one of the genes the baby received from his parents. It is one of the most common reasons children become mentally disabled in the United States. Down syndrome affects one out of every 700 to 1,000 babies born each year.

Edward's syndrome

This is also a chromosome problem. Babies born with Edward's syndrome have small heads and often have a cleft palate. Their hearts and digestive systems may not be formed properly. Most die in the first year of their lives.

Turner's syndrome

Only girls are born with Turner's syndrome. They have a distinctive appearance, a little like a baby with Down syndrome. But these children often are not mentally disabled. They may have heart problems. Their genital organs do not develop properly, and they are often sterile.

Spina bifida

This condition means that the bones of the baby's spine do not protect his spinal cord properly. Spina bifida can be very serious. Affected persons may be paralyzed and lack bladder or bowel control. Or the condition may be mild and cause the person no problems at all during his life.

Anencephaly

This means the baby's brain and skull have not developed as they should. Affected babies can only live for a few minutes or hours after birth.

Cleft lip and/or palate

In the uterus, the baby's mouth develops in two parts, which then join together. Sometimes the parts do not join and the baby is born with a hole in his lip or the roof of his mouth. Surgery for these conditions is now excellent. Cleft lips are treated as early as 3 to 4 months of age. Cleft palates can be closed during the second year of the baby's life.

age. We discussed what would happen if the result was positive, and how and when an abortion could be performed. She also sent me written information."

There are now so many tests that it helps to sort out which tests, if any, you want to have. Many tests are only valid if they are given at a certain time in pregnancy. Thus you need to plan them almost as soon as you know you are pregnant: *"I saw my doctor when I was 5 weeks pregnant just so I could figure out the 'right' tests for me and when to have them."*

If You Have a Positive Result from a Prenatal Test

- Ask at once to speak to a doctor or nurse.
- Ask if you can speak with a prenatal screening counselor. In some places, nurses with special training are on hand to offer information and support while you make the choices you need to make.
- Find out exactly what the result means.
- Find out what your options are.
- Ask to be given contact names for groups with a special knowledge of the condition your baby may have. Talk to your partner or friends or anyone who will listen to you carefully about the result of the test and what you are going to do next.
- Give yourself time in which to decide.
- Remember that it's *all right* to change your mind.

Either the mother or the father of the child may have very strong feelings about testing. These may be based upon what they have read, heard or experienced, or upon their feelings about having a child with disabilities. The couple may agree to act upon the feelings of one of them. But it is still important that they do this only after learning all they can:

"When I got pregnant, Matt said his first wife had had an amniocentesis because of her age. He more or less insisted that I have one. I just went along with it, without even thinking what might happen if there was anything wrong. Now I wish I'd thought more about it."

"We talked about not having the tests. But Mark finally went along with me because I'm the one who stays at home. He would still have to deal with being the father of a child with disabilities. But I would be the one doing most of the day-to-day care."

Choosing not to have tests

Some women choose, early in their pregnancies, not to have any tests at all. This may be because they wouldn't think of having an abortion even if something was wrong with the baby. Or they might find the risks of the tests to be much higher than the risk of the baby having a serious problem:

"I asked not to have the tests. My midwife had just assumed that I would. She asked how old I was and then she said, 'Well, I assume you'll be wanting the tests.' I said, 'Well, no, I don't want to.' Even after I'd said

that, she asked when she was taking blood, 'Shall I take enough in case you decide that you do want the screening test?' There's a lot of pressure on you to have the test. The problem is I know that I couldn't do anything about a result that was abnormal. I know I couldn't have an abortion."

"We've decided not to have any screening at all. A friend of ours had the triple-screen test and came out with a 1 in 49 chance of having a child with Down syndrome. But when the baby was born, he was fine. She had to go through all that trauma about whether or not to have an amniocentesis and whether or not she'd have an abortion. So we're not going to have any screening."

The choice not to have testing may also be made because of earlier tragedies in the couple's life: *"I don't want any tests. I don't think I could have an abortion if there was something wrong. I've lost two babies. I couldn't possibly abort this one."*

Tests You Can Choose
Chorionic villus sampling (CVS)

The earliest test a woman can choose to have is CVS, or chorionic villus sampling. For most women, the value of this test is that it can be done early in pregnancy. Then, if the result is abnormal, the pregnancy can be brought to an end at an early stage: *"I had CVS. I was eager to have it. I asked to have it. I think I would have been offered it anyway because of my age. Where I live it's routine to offer it to women who will be over 35 when they give birth. I wanted to have it because you can have it sooner in pregnancy than an amniocentesis. I thought if there were a problem and I did decide to abort, at least it would be as early as possible. I had the test at 12 weeks."*

How a woman copes with prenatal testing depends to a large extent on the support she receives: *"I was well counseled beforehand by a nurse. I felt positive about it."*

When you understand what is happening, the procedure itself is much more bearable: *"The procedure wasn't fun. But it also wasn't as bad as I'd expected. I felt it was handled very well. I felt really well informed. And I had the results within 48 hours. They phoned me at home."*

Chorionic Villus Sampling (CVS)

Type of test: DIAGNOSTIC

When is it done?

Around 11 weeks

What conditions is it looking for?

Down syndrome
Turner's syndrome
Edward's syndrome
(*not* spina bifida)

How is it done?

The doctor passes a fine needle either through the wall of your abdomen, or into the vagina and through the cervix. An ultrasound scan is used to help find the placenta so that a very small piece of it may be sucked out through the needle. The procedure isn't pleasant. But it's not normally painful, either. It takes from 10 to 20 minutes and is done in the outpatient clinic of your local hospital.

How long before the results come back?

7-10 days

If the result is abnormal, what next?

You could choose:

– To do nothing

– To end your pregnancy (have an abortion)

Research shows that more women miscarry after having CVS than after amniocentesis. Some women who are old enough to be at increased risk of having a baby with Down syndrome decide against the CVS test for this reason: *"I chose to have an amnio rather than CVS because of the risks involved. The hospital we're near seems to have fewer miscarriages after amnio than CVS. At least that's what we were told."*

Miscarriage rates for both CVS and amniocentesis are lower when the procedures are performed by doctors who do a lot of them each year, rather than by doctors who only do a few. Seek out a specialist if you can afford one, or if your health plan will cover the cost. It will be safer for the baby than it would be if these tests were performed by someone who has had less practice at it.

There have been some reports that having CVS very early in pregnancy, before 11 weeks, may cause the baby to be born with abnormal arms and legs. Although CVS is now performed later than it used to be, some couples remain anxious that there may still be a risk of their baby being hurt by the test: *"We were offered CVS and were told about the risk of miscarriage— 2%. The risk of the test being wrong was also 2%. And, most important to us, there was a chance it might damage the baby. We chose amnio-centesis instead."*

The choice to have or not to have CVS is a personal one. There are no absolute rights or wrongs about prenatal testing. The choice to have a test can only be based on each woman's views after she becomes informed and weighs the test's positive and negative features.

Blood tests

The AFP test measures the level of alpha-fetoprotein in a sample of the mother's blood. The double-screen test measures AFP and also the level of the hormone human chorionic gonadotrophin. The triple-screen test measures the first two plus blood levels of the hormone estriol. These blood tests assess the risk of the mother carrying a baby with Down syndrome, spina bifida and some other conditions. Be aware that these are screening tests. The results of these tests are not conclusive. These tests aim to let you know how much at risk you are of having a baby with disabilities. You can use the results from these tests to make other decisions about testing:

"I paid to have the triple-screen test done. I also arranged for an amniocentesis because I was over 37. The triple-screen test results were

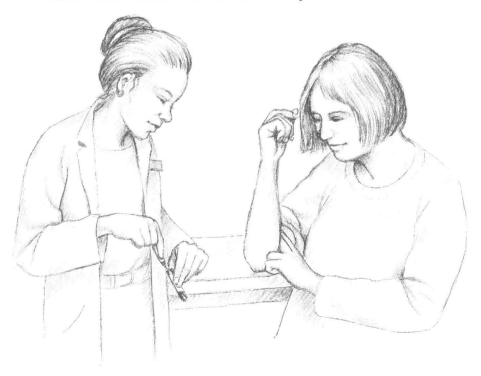

The Double-Screen or Triple-Screen Test

Type of test: SCREENING

When is it done?
15 to 18 weeks

What conditions is it looking for?
Down syndrome
Spina bifida
Anencephaly
Turner's syndrome
Edward's syndrome
and some other rare conditions

How is it done?
By taking a small amount of blood from your arm.

Some of these tests are offered to all pregnant women. Some are only offered to women over 30 or 35 who are at increased risk of having a baby with Down syndrome. If you are under 30 and want to have a test, *ask*. You will almost certainly be able to have it.

The triple-screen test looks at three different markers in the mother's blood to assess the risk of her baby having Down syndrome. The double-screen test looks at two different markers.

How long before the results come back?
48 hours

If the result is abnormal, what next?
You could choose:

– To do nothing

– To have a "high-resolution" ultrasound scan. This is used to check the baby's spine if your baby is thought to be at risk of spina bifida

– To have an amniocentesis

good for my age, so I canceled the amnio."

"When I first went to the hospital, I was given a leaflet about the AFP test. I decided that since there was no risk to the baby with the test, I might as well have it done. Depending on the results, I'd decide what to do next. Even if the result were positive, I might not do anything else. I know sometimes the test shows positive even when the baby is all right."

Even when the woman is at very low risk of having a baby with Down syndrome or any other problem, waiting for the result can be nerve-racking: *"They said ten days until the result comes back. You count the days. And when ten days have gone, you start thinking it must be OK. You're sitting there during those ten days and each time the phone rings, you're thinking, 'Well, I wonder if that's the hospital calling?'"*

Often you are contacted only if the AFP result is abnormal. If the result is higher than average, your baby may be at risk of spina bifida. If it's lower than average, your baby may have Down syndrome. You often hear nothing if the test is within normal limits. This can be upsetting: *"It would be nice to have a letter telling you the result's normal. Otherwise you're thinking, 'Well, is my test mixed up with someone else's?' I'd like a letter in my hand to say the test's been done and it's OK."*

After getting the news of an abnormal result, some women find they have to endure more waiting until they can see a doctor with whom they can discuss what to do next: *"A nurse phoned on Friday and told us something might be wrong with the baby. She told us nothing more. We spent the weekend going crazy. We tried to find out what having a high AFP result meant. I went to the hospital on Monday morning. The nurse there told me I was at risk of having a baby with spina bifida. I still had to wait to see a doctor. That took another two hours."*

"When I was 16 weeks pregnant, I had a double-screen test. About two weeks later, a nurse phoned and said she had some bad news. She told me I needed to go to the hospital the next day for an amniocentesis. I tried to question her, but all she would add was that my baby was at risk of Down syndrome. She said I could talk to a doctor at the hospital. Needless to say, I was frantic for 24 hours."

Some women live to regret having had the AFP test. An abnormal result puts a doubt in their minds as to whether or not the baby is healthy. If the baby is suspected of having spina bifida, you may choose to have a high-resolution ultrasound scan. This can confirm (or deny) the suspicion. It is safer than having an amniocentesis, which carries a risk that the baby will miscarry. If the baby is suspected of having Down syndrome, amniocentesis lets you know for sure. But some women do not want to choose amniocentesis. That's because, if the result is positive, it leads to a decision about ending the pregnancy:

"I was very upset when I got the bad news about the AFP. I spent a sleepless night running through the options about amniocentesis and whether I'd have an abortion. I remembered vividly from my days as a nurse how really upsetting late abortions are. I knew I would have to be very convinced of the baby having a serious problem before I could endure one. I wished I'd never had the AFP test. But I hadn't considered these matters in advance."

A blood test that comes back "screen positive" and states the woman's risk of having a baby with Down syndrome can be very hard to understand: *"If you know that you have a baby with Down syndrome, that's very different from being told you've got a 1 in 48 chance of having one."*

Blood Tests for Prenatal Screening

A pregnant woman's blood can be tested to see whether her baby has any of several conditions. But blood tests are mainly used to detect spina bifida and Down syndrome. Down syndrome is one of the most common causes of serious mental problems.

Young women are at lower risk of having a baby with Down syndrome than older women. At the age of 20, your chance of having a baby with Down syndrome is about 1 in 1700. At the age of 45, your chance is 1 in 30.

Blood tests are used to better assess your risk. You may be told that the risk of having a Down baby at your age is 1 in 200, but the risk based on your blood test is 1 in 350. This means that you are at a much smaller risk of having a baby with Down syndrome than most women your age.

But if your risk, based on your age, is 1 in 500, and your risk based on your blood test is 1 in 60, you are at much higher risk of having a baby with Down syndrome than other women your age.

Most hospitals use a cutoff point of a risk of 1 in 250. This means that if your risk is less than 1 in 250, your blood test will be described as "screen negative." If your risk is greater than 1 in 250, your test will be described as "screen positive." So, the fact that your test is screen negative doesn't mean for certain that your baby does not have Down syndrome. And the fact that you are screen positive doesn't mean that your baby actually has Down syndrome.

The risk of a baby having spina bifida is not related to the mother's age. It can be related to prenatal exposure of either parent to toxic agents. There is also evidence that adequate folic acid in the mother's diet, before conception and early in pregnancy, can help protect against spina bifida. About 1 in every 2000 babies born has spina bifida. But spina bifida isn't always serious. Some children with spina bifida have hardly any problems. But others will need to be in a wheelchair with 24-hour-a-day care.

AFP (Alpha-fetoprotein)

Type of test: SCREENING

When is it done?

15-18 weeks

How long before the results come back?

About 10 days (often women are only told if the result is positive)

What conditions is it looking for?

Spina bifida
Down syndrome
Turner's syndrome

How is it done?

By taking a small amount of blood from your arm

If the result is positive, what next?

You could choose:

– To do nothing

– To have a "high resolution" ultrasound scan. This is used to check the baby's spine if your baby is thought to be at risk of spina bifida

– To have an amniocentesis

The first decision, to have a screening test, now leads to another—whether to have an amniocentesis. With this test you can be certain of whether the baby has Down syndrome or other serious problems. But it can be an unpleasant procedure for the woman and risky for the baby. It also means three weeks of waiting for the result. If the result comes back positive, you have to make another choice right away. Will you continue or end the pregnancy? It can seem that where prenatal testing is concerned, small decisions lead to ever-harder ones.

Amniocentesis

Some women choose not to have any blood tests but simply go straight for an amniocentesis: *"I didn't really trust the AFP. I've known people for whom the result has been normal, and they've had children with Down syndrome or spina bifida. So I asked for an amnio. It reassured me. The results take quite a while. But I wasn't too upset during that time since I didn't think of myself as high risk. I didn't mind waiting."*

A fear of the extra commitment that comes with having a baby with Down syndrome spurs some women to choose amniocentesis even though they know the test could cause a miscarriage: *"I was prepared to have an amniocentesis. I felt that if I had a child with Down syndrome, that would be the end of my life, my work and my marriage, too. I didn't want to have one because I've seen two or three people with Down children whose lives have fallen apart."*

A healthcare provider's view of a woman's risk of having a baby with Down syndrome may not be the same as her own: *"My doctor told me the risk of Down syndrome for my age group was 1 in 300. She said that in her view this was not a large risk. I didn't agree. So I went ahead and asked for amniocentesis."*

A woman may feel pressure to state that she is certain she will have an abortion if the amniocentesis result is positive. Some women have no doubt that they would choose to end the pregnancy if their baby were diagnosed with Down syndrome. Others simply want to know for certain so they can have time to prepare themselves for the birth of a baby with special needs: *"I was told that an amniocentesis could only be performed if I planned to abort if the results were positive. I argued that I wanted to know if I was having a baby with Down syndrome so that I could prepare for its arrival. So they went ahead and performed the*

Amniocentesis

Type of test: DIAGNOSTIC

When is it done?

16 to 18 weeks

(but soon the test may be offered much earlier in pregnancy)

What conditions is it looking for?

Down syndrome
Edward's syndrome
Turner's syndrome
Spina bifida
Anencephaly
and other rare conditions

How is it done?

A fine needle is put through the wall of your abdomen using ultrasound as a guide. The doctor takes a sample of the fluid (waters) that surround the baby. This fluid contains cells from the baby. These are sent to a lab. The procedure takes from 10 to 20 minutes to carry out. It can be done at most hospitals in the outpatient department.

How long before the results come back?

3 to 4 weeks

If the test is positive, what next?

You could choose:

– To do nothing

– To end your pregnancy
(have an abortion)

amnio without a decision about an abortion."

Some women resist the pressure to discuss abortion before the amniocentesis by seeming to go along with the wishes of the doctor or clinic: *"My doctor made it clear that it was only worth my having an amniocentesis if we would go for an abortion. I said, 'Fine,' although I hadn't really decided. I reserved the right to decide later and say, 'Sorry, I'm going ahead with my pregnancy.'"*

There should be no pressure on the woman about abortion one way or the other: *"I chose not to think about abortion before the amnio. The doctor said it was a 'good attitude.'"*

Having an amniocentesis can be very different for different women. The difference may depend on how worried the woman is about the outcome: *"I wanted to have an amniocentesis so I could be reassured. I'm not at high risk of having a baby with Down syndrome because I'm only 27. The amnio was OK. It wasn't painful or anything. I just felt a push as the needle went in."*

"I was almost 36 when I conceived. My husband and I had already discussed having an amnio. Lee was with me throughout the test. I didn't really expect to feel as shocked as I did afterward. The feeling of contraction as the needle goes in and comes out was very strange, although I had been warned to expect it. I was told to rest for 24 hours afterward. I was in shock for at least a day."

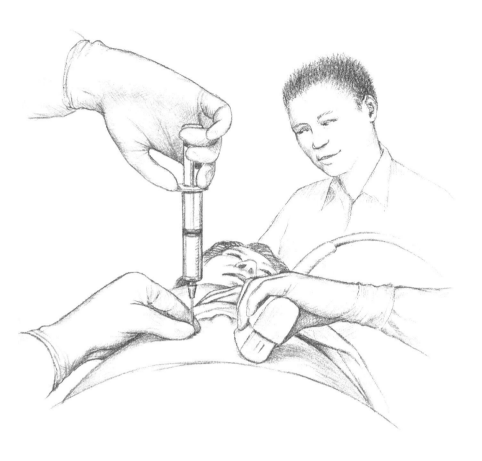

The procedure for taking two samples of fluid in a twin pregnancy can take longer and be more difficult: *"They extracted the fluid from around the first baby with no problem. But there was a membrane in the way of the second and they couldn't get any [fluid from there]. I was there for hours with a few rests [between attempts]. In the end, they had to call in the senior doctor, who finally got it. But I had had the needle inserted in a number of places across my belly."*

Although the chance of miscarriage is small after an amniocentesis, the risk exists. There are times when prenatal testing leads to a series of events that change the woman's life forever: *"I was not counseled about the AFP test. I accepted it as routine. I was 20 weeks pregnant when I was told that, although I was only 26, I had the risk of a woman of 37 of having a baby with Down syndrome. The amnio was set up for the*

Pros and Cons of Prenatal Tests

Test	Pros	Cons
CVS (chorionic villus sampling)	Carried out early in pregnancy. An abortion, if needed, is simple to perform. It may be easier for the mother to cope with when it is done so early in pregnancy.	Risk of miscarriage—The chance of this depends in part on the skill of the person who performs the test. Ask your doctor about his rate of miscarriage following CVS (it will probably be about 2%). May not be obtained at all hospitals.
Alpha-fetoprotein	A simple blood test that carries no risk to the baby.	Not too reliable. Most women who are told they are at high risk— 19 out of 20—will NOT have a baby with spina bifida.
Double-screen test/Triple-screen test	A simple blood test that carries no risk to the baby.	Can be very hard to know whether to have more tests if your risk comes back as higher than average. After all, even a 1-in-5 risk of having a baby with Down syndrome still means that you are far more likely *not* to have an affected baby.
Amniocentesis	Gives you a definite result.	Risk of miscarriage afterwards— Ask your doctor what his rate is (it will probably be 1% to 2%). Carried out fairly late in pregnancy (16 to 18 weeks). You have to wait 3 or 4 weeks for the result. If you decide to abort, you will be well along in pregnancy and will have to go through labor.
Ultrasound scans	Can give all sorts of information about the health of the baby. You can see your baby on the screen. Can be carried out at any point in pregnancy.	The usefulness of the scan depends on: (a) how good the sonographer is at reading the scan (b) how good the scanning equipment is (c) how long you are scanned

There is a shortage of long-term research into ultrasound. It may have effects on unborn babies that we don't know yet. |

next day. I had no time at all to think it over. I was single and really stressed. I had the amnio on Tuesday, and the next Friday I started getting pains that I now know were the start of labor. I went to the hospital that night and gave birth to a little girl six hours later. I was not told of the results of the amnio until I called the hospital. Then they told me that the baby had been normal. This was all nearly four years ago. I am still mourning the loss of my daughter. She would have been just about ready to go to school now had it not been for the prenatal testing."

About 1 in 100 women miscarry after having an amniocentesis. But this statistic varies with the skill of the doctor who performs the test. Doctors who perform the test more often tend to have lower miscarriage rates. So it makes sense to shop around for a specialist who does a lot of prenatal testing, if you can. Ask about the doctor's miscarriage rate before you sign up for the test.

Waiting for the results of an amniocentesis may take up to four weeks. The time can seem endless when so much may depend on the outcome: *"If the result had been positive, my doctor would've phoned right away. So for at least the last week of the three weeks' wait, I went nuts each time the phone rang."*

A negative result can provide a great deal of comfort. It may enable the woman to relax and enjoy the rest of her pregnancy. But it doesn't always work that way:

"My friend had the AFP test, which was slightly low. Then she had an amnio and things were fine and normal. But she still couldn't stop worrying. It didn't comfort her. She worried for the rest of her pregnancy. So for her it didn't work."

"Having an amnio and waiting for the results changed my whole attitude towards the baby. The last few months of my pregnancy were frightening. I was still worried even after I'd gotten the negative result. Now I'm planning my second pregnancy. I really don't know whether to have any tests this time."

A positive result leads you to decide whether or not to end the pregnancy. Some women feel strongly before the amniocentesis that they would have an abortion if Down syndrome were diagnosed. But they may feel uncertain when it comes down to making the actual choice: *"The baby's got Down syndrome. But I don't know how badly the baby is affected. It could be a mild case."*

Other people can make a difference: *"We had a friend whose daughter had spina bifida. She died when she was twelve. He said to me one day last year: 'If my wife and I had known, we would not have had her. Although we loved her, she had no life at all.' That made a very strong impression on me."*

When a woman is thinking about ending her pregnancy, she needs good counseling from healthcare providers. She can also turn to other women who have had to make the same decision or to a minister, priest or rabbi. There are also groups that help parents who are thinking about an abortion or that can help them understand what is involved in caring for a child with disabilities:

"I contacted the National Down Syndrome Society, which sent me some things to read. I also got in touch with the local college. It works with the National Down Syndrome Society. I went to see their work with children with Down syndrome and their families."

If a woman has a twin pregnancy and one baby is found to be normal but the other has Down syndrome, she could choose to carry out what is called "selective abortion" and abort just one baby:

"The obstetrician was very kind. He talked with us and gave us lots of time. There was a small risk of miscarriage. But we knew without doubt that we wanted to go ahead. We had to put our faith in him and his great reputation. But I couldn't help thinking that night, 'What if they get the wrong baby?' We went back the next day for the abortion. The baby's heart was injected and it just took an instant. Right afterwards, they showed me the other baby moving about, unaffected. I was very upset. I had to sweat it out for three more days. At last they phoned me with the results of a blood sample they had taken from the aborted baby to say that yes, the baby had Down syndrome. For the rest of my pregnancy, I worried about the other baby."

The choice not to abort may be made on moral or religious grounds. Or perhaps the woman doesn't believe that having a baby with disabilities is such a terrible thing. Or she may want to know and care for her baby, however briefly. A midwife remembers a couple who chose to have their baby in spite of the fact that it was not expected to survive: *"The amniocentesis came back that the baby had a really serious condition. They decided not to abort. They went on to have a normal labor. And yes, the baby was clearly not going to survive. But they got to hold the baby and the baby died in her arms. She felt that this was how it should be. They could give the baby the comfort of their arms and get something back themselves."*

Ultrasound scanning

When ultrasound scanning in pregnancy was first introduced in the United States, there was a great deal of excitement among women and their doctors. Scans were done, in some cases, weekly, throughout pregnancy. Since those early days, more restraint has been exercised. Now, routine scanning may consist of two scans only. One may be done at about 12 weeks to date the pregnancy. Another may be done to look for problems in the baby at about 18 weeks. Some well-informed people are starting to urge even greater caution in the use of scanning. They warn that little long-term research has been done into

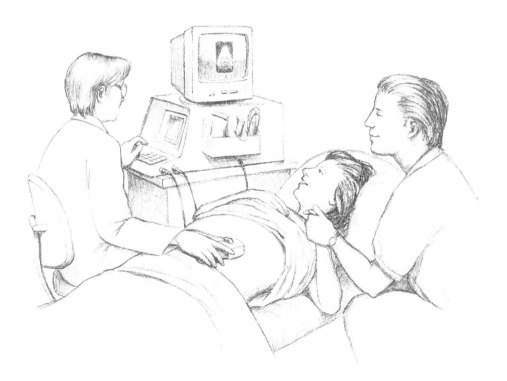

Ultrasound Scans in Pregnancy

Nuchal Test

Type of test: SCREENING

When is it done?

10 to 13 weeks (May only be obtained from specialists)

What condition is it looking for?

Down syndrome

How is it done?

You have an ultrasound scan. The doctor or technician measures the amount of fluid beneath the skin behind the baby's neck. This measurement can indicate the chance of the baby having Down syndrome.

How long before the results come back?

Right away

If the test is positive, what next?

You could choose:

– To do nothing

– To have CVS (chorionic villus sampling)

– To have a blood test (AFP or the double-screen or triple-screen test)

– To have amniocentesis

Fetal-Anomaly Scan

Type of Test: SCREENING

When is it done?

18 to 20 weeks

What conditions is it looking for?

A range of disorders. The scan checks the baby's arms and legs, spine, heart, brain and kidneys.

Spina bifida
Anencephaly
Cleft lip and palate

How is it done?

A cold, jelly-like substance is put on your abdomen. Then the technician passes a transducer across your abdomen and looks at the picture of the baby on a screen. You will be able to see the image too. The technician will point out your baby's face, hands and feet.

How long before the results come back?

Right away

If the scan shows a problem, what next?

You could choose:

– To do nothing

– To have another, more detailed scan

– To have amniocentesis

A high-resolution ultrasound scan is extremely detailed. It uses a very expensive scanner. Such scans may reveal spina bifida in a baby. In this case, ultrasound becomes a diagnostic test rather than a screening test.

its possible effects on children. One Norwegian study suggested that scanning led to an increase in the number of left-handed children. The researchers felt that this might be due to changes in the way the brain develops brought about by ultrasound.

As with all the other forms of testing discussed above, women have their own views about ultrasound. They have the right to make up their own minds: *"I thought the scan was wonderful. The baby looked as if it was moving around."*

"It's helped me and my partner bond with the baby."

"It's almost as if the procedure is there, so we have to use it. I don't agree with that."

Some people are alarmed by recent negative TV and newspaper reports about ultrasound scans in pregnancy. These reports can confuse parents: *"Each time I read something about the dangers of ultrasound, I read something else that says the total opposite. Nothing's been proved. It's very hard to make a decision."*

Women can find themselves under a lot of pressure to follow the routine care provided by the hospital: *"They were coming around and were almost abusive in the end because I would not have an ultrasound. I kept saying, 'I'm sorry, I will not have one. I do not want to have one. This is my body and my decision. I've weighed all the pros and cons, and I do not want an ultrasound.' And the nurses kept saying, 'The doctor's getting very upset because you won't.' The emotional blackmail was amazing."*

If the baby is seen on the screen during an early scan, a miscarriage can be even harder to cope with: *"It almost made it harder, seeing that Lydia was OK, moving around, and hearing the heartbeat. And then I lost her five weeks later."*

On the other hand, an ultrasound image may become part of the healing process after a miscarriage: *"Although it upset me seeing the baby on scan and then his dying, at least I saw him, and it made him real. With the scan, we have a lasting picture. And that's all we've got. So that's really important."*

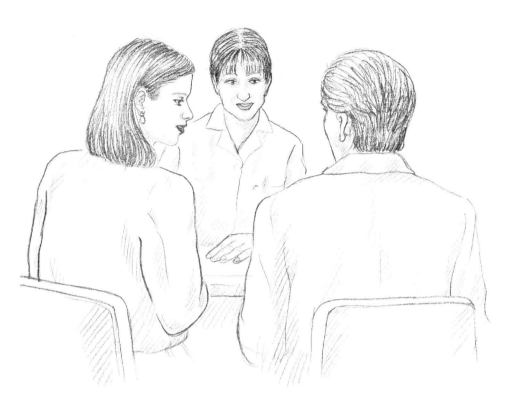

Informed Choice

The pressures created by prenatal testing are immense. The choices that have to be made are complex. You have to decide whether to have a certain test and then about what to do if the test is positive. These are choices that can be made only by the woman herself. Women's feelings about testing differ a great deal. What is right for one woman is not right for another. Finding your way through the maze of tests is not easy. But it seems that women feel better about these choices when they have been fully informed.

You need to know what your options are. And you may need help thinking about what you will do if test results are positive. A woman needs to be informed and to be given time to make her decision without pressure. Then, chances are she will feel content about the tests she decides to have:

"I felt the nurse had discussed everything I needed to know at the time to make a decision. She stressed that whatever I decided, I could change my mind. I saw her again later and we discussed my decision. She gave me a date for the test, told me what would happen and how I would learn about the result. She also gave me a phone number if I wanted to learn more. The counseling helped me make an informed choice."

Blood Tests in Pregnancy

When you have your first prenatal visit, the nurse will take some blood from your arm for routine testing:

1. To find out your blood group
2. To find out whether you are Rhesus negative
3. To check your hemoglobin level (whether you're anemic)
4. To test for syphilis (sexually transmitted disease)
5. To see if you are immune to rubella (German measles)
6. To test for blood problems such as:
   – sickle-cell anemia, which is common among people of West Indian and African descent
   – thalassemia, which is common among people of Mediterranean descent

Blood samples for hemoglobin testing may be taken again at:
   – 28 weeks and 36 weeks of pregnancy

If you are Rh-negative, you may have additional blood tests at:
   – 28, 32, 36 and 40 weeks of pregnancy

Testing for HIV (AIDS)

In some places, the blood of all pregnant women is routinely tested for HIV, but the testing is anonymous. That means the result cannot be traced back to you.

The test should not be done without your consent. If you want to know if this is happening, ask the doctor or nurse who takes blood from you at your first prenatal visit.

If you think you might like to have an HIV test, ask to discuss the matter with a counselor, your doctor or your midwife. All hospitals should provide counseling from someone with training in HIV issues.

It's important to think carefully about the pros and cons before having a test.

What Happens in a Blood Test

Rhesus factor

Some women are described as having Rhesus-negative (or Rh-negative) blood. This can be a problem if the baby has Rh-positive blood. During the birth, blood cells from the baby can pass into the mother's bloodstream. The mother's body reacts to the foreign blood cells by making antibodies to destroy them. If the mother becomes pregnant again with a Rhesus-positive baby, these antibodies will pass to the baby and start to destroy his red blood cells.

So after giving birth, each Rh-negative mother is given a shot of a protective blood product (trade name RhoGAM®). This masks any of the baby's red blood cells that have gotten into her bloodstream. Once this has been done, the mother's body does not make antibodies against them.

Women who are Rh-negative have their blood tested more often during pregnancy to make sure that they are not forming antibodies. If antibodies are found, the baby can be treated with blood transfusions while still in the uterus.

Nowadays, Rh-negative women don't have problems if they have good prenatal care during each of their pregnancies.

Rubella testing

If your blood sample shows that you are not immune to rubella:

1. You will be advised to keep away from any child or adult who may have rubella (German measles).

2. You will be advised to get a vaccine against rubella once your baby has been born. (You need to make sure you won't get pregnant for the next three months!)

3. If your blood sample shows that you have been infected with rubella recently, you will be offered an abortion. This is offered because there is a very high risk of the baby being born with serious problems.

Anemia

If your blood tests show that you have low levels of hemoglobin, you may:

1. Be advised to eat more foods such as bread, cereals and potatoes, which are rich in iron. You may also be asked to eat more fruit and vegetables that contain vitamin C to help your body absorb iron.

2. Be prescribed iron supplements. (These work best when they are taken with the first and last meal of the day.)

All pregnant women appear to be slightly anemic because their blood is thinner than that of nonpregnant women. They have the same amount of red blood cells, but the blood cells are much more diluted in the bloodstream. There is a strong feeling that mild anemia in pregnancy should not be treated. It is felt that thinner blood may circulate better through the placenta.

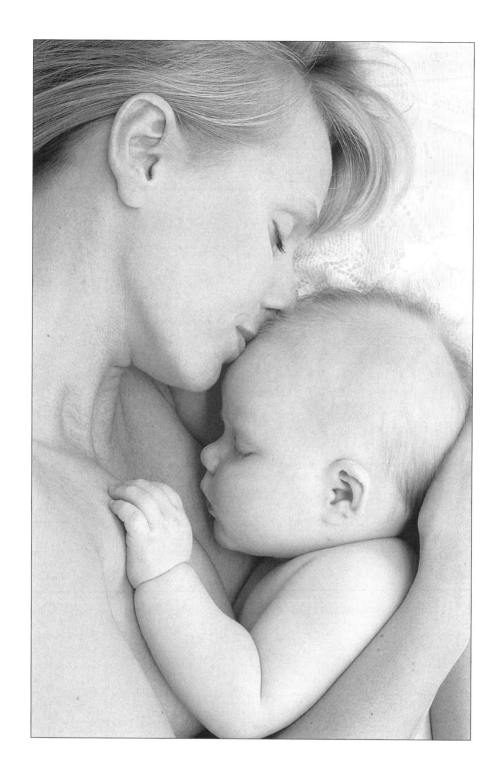

CHAPTER 4 *What Labor Is Like*

No matter how many women you talk to about what happened to them during their labor, one thing is certain. Your labor will be different from any of theirs. That does not mean you can't learn a lot about birth from other mothers; you can. Certain things happen in all normal labors. Contractions or labor pains open the neck of the womb until it is wide enough for the baby to pass through (about ten centimeters [cm]). Then the womb and the mother both push the baby out into the world. Finally the placenta or afterbirth is born. But many variations exist, even within this basic framework. It would be unwise to think that because you have read all the books and been to lots of classes that you know exactly what is going to happen to you.

The Three Stages of Labor

Labor is divided into three stages:

First Stage

Contractions make the cervix or neck of the womb open from 0cm to about 10cm in the first stage. Your progress is checked by how many centimeters your cervix has dilated. If you are having your first baby, first stage may last from 12 to 18 hours.

Second Stage

This is the "pushing" part of labor, when you give birth to your baby. It often lasts about two hours for a first baby. But some women find it takes less than 20 minutes.

Third Stage

After the baby has been born, the placenta needs to come out of the uterus. This happens in the third stage of labor. Third stage can last a few minutes or more than an hour (see third-stage box, page 88).

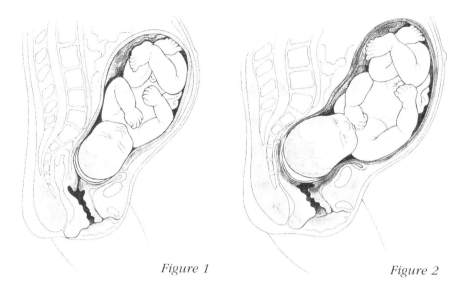

Figure 1   *Figure 2*

Figures 1 through 4 show how the cervix (the neck of the womb) opens during the first stage of labor. The baby moves lower into the mother's pelvis. Meanwhile his head turns so that his face is toward her spine. This is the position in which it is easiest for him to be born. You can see how the bag of waters bulges in front of the baby's head toward the end of the first stage (figure 4). The waters often break at this time.

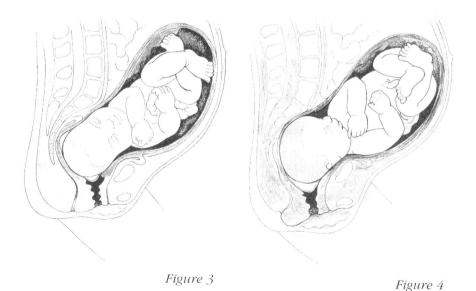

Figure 3

Figure 4

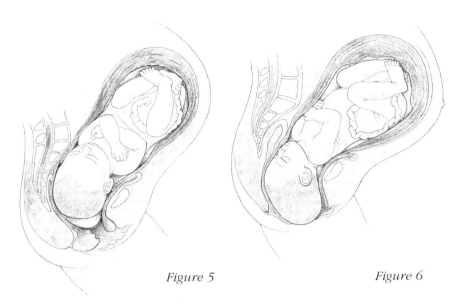

Figure 5   *Figure 6*

When the cervix is open as wide as it needs to be for the baby to come through (about 10cm), the uterus and the mother push the baby out of the pelvis (figures 5 through 7). The baby is working hard to be born, too. He untucks his head and stretches his neck so he can move around the mother's pubic bone and out of the vagina. After his head has been born, the baby turns his head to help bring his shoulders out of the vagina (figure 8). His whole body will be born with the next contraction.

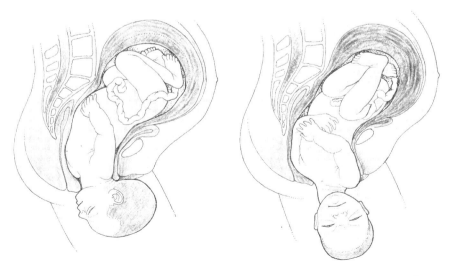

Figure 7   *Figure 8*

Feeling in Control

Many pregnant women talk about how important it will be for them to feel in control of their labor. But during parts of your labor you may feel out of control. The contractions can become extremely strong and powerful. You may feel taken over by them. There may be moments when it seems the birth of your baby will never happen. You may feel you will never get to that magical moment when she is finally placed in your arms. It's hard to feel in control at times like these.

It helps to understand what's going on. You'll feel better if you know how far along in labor you are and if your baby is OK. If your contractions are coming so fast that you can't ask questions yourself, your labor-support person can ask for you. Then he or she can tell you. Labor-support people are often better than health providers at speaking with women in strong labor because they know them so well.

Feeling in control is not about not shouting or swearing or tearing off your nightgown because you're too hot. It's about your midwife or labor-support person talking with you. This person needs to keep you informed. He or she also needs to encourage and reassure you. Not being spoken to leads to feelings of panic. *"The more they rushed around and didn't tell me what was going on, the more I panicked. They kept telling my husband to leave the room. He didn't know what was going on, either. He was very frightened."*

When communication has been good in labor, most women feel pleased with their care. It doesn't matter what course the events of labor have taken. *"The nurses gave me so much confidence in myself. They listened to what I wanted. It really helped to have faith in my own body. I felt it was doing what it was meant to do. I'm glad I've gone through labor."*

The start of labor

During pregnancy, women and their partners are often very anxious about how they will know when labor has started. It helps to understand labor doesn't have a certain starting point—it's not as if you're pregnant one minute and then in labor the next. The neck of the uterus, the cervix, changes over a number of days in the early part of

Am I in Labor?

You have had a "show"

This means the small plug of mucus, which sealed the neck of the uterus (cervix) during pregnancy, has dropped out. The cervix is starting to soften and open. It's a very early sign of labor. You need to stay calm and wait for something else.

WHAT'S OK
The show is jelly-like and slightly pink because it is streaked with a little blood.

WHAT'S NOT OK
The show should not come with a sudden loss of blood similar to your period. If you are losing blood freely, contact your doctor, midwife or the hospital right away.

Your waters have broken

Call the doctor or midwife who is going to help you give birth and ask for advice. You will be asked these questions:

• When do you think your waters broke?

• Did they go with a gush or did you simply notice your underwear was damp?

• What color is the fluid you are losing?

• What does it smell like?

• Have you had a show?

• Are you having any contractions?

WHAT'S OK
The waters are clear or straw-colored.

WHAT'S NOT OK
They should not be green-brown in color or bad-smelling. If they are

muddy, this means that your baby has moved his bowels in the uterus. This is often (but not always) a sign that he is distressed and may need to be born quickly.

You are having contractions

Contractions may be your first sign that labor has started. Women don't always notice they've had a show. Most of the time the waters don't break until labor is far along. It's not always easy to know from the contractions how far along you are in labor. Ask yourself the following questions. Don't hesitate to contact your doctor or midwife if you aren't sure what to do.

ASK YOURSELF:

• When did the contractions start?

• How long are they lasting now?

• How often are they coming?

• How painful are they?

(This question may be hard to answer. Ask yourself whether you can still talk or work while having an episode. Do you need to stop to lean on something and focus on your breathing?)

• Am I happy coping on my own or with my labor-support person?

• Would I prefer to have a nurse or midwife with me?

If the answer to the last question is "yes," phone your midwife and ask her to come to you if you are having a home birth. Or go to the hospital after letting the maternity ward know when you will arrive.

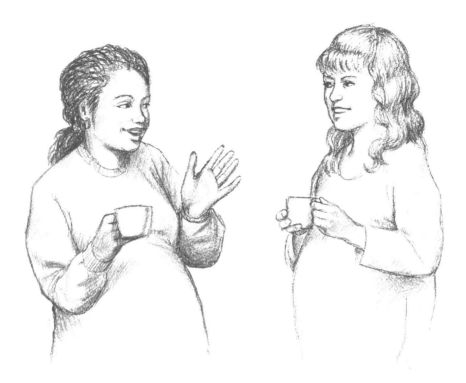

labor. It goes from being long and firm like the tip of the nose, to shorter and softer—more like the texture of the lips. You might not be aware that anything is happening. Or you may have a few days of bothersome, period-like pains. After a while it becomes clear that you are in labor and your baby is coming. There may be a show when the plug of mucus, which has sealed the cervix during pregnancy, drops out. Or the waters may break. Or the contractions may begin to make themselves felt.

"I had a show when I was getting out of the shower. It was obvious. I knew right away what it was."

"I'd had a few days of what I thought were Braxton-Hicks contractions. They were few and far between. Then I was lying in bed, reading a book, and I heard this 'pop' and my waters broke. There was a lot of fluid, which surprised me."

"I'd invited a friend to come over for the afternoon. While we were talking, I began to have contractions. I knew they were the real thing even

though they didn't hurt much. I kept on talking to Melanie while I was having them. I didn't tell her I had started labor. We kept talking, and I walked her out to her car, which was parked down the street, contracting every 10 minutes."

Labor gets started slowly as the amount of oxytocin, the hormone that causes contractions, builds up in your body. Contractions don't start "out of the blue." Ever since you were a baby yourself, growing in your mother's womb, your uterus has been contracting. (If the baby you are pregnant with is a little girl, her womb is contracting inside you, too.) But you haven't been aware of it unless you've suffered from painful period cramps. During your pregnancy, you may have been surprised that, sometimes, your tummy gets very hard, like a rock. This is your womb contracting, getting ready for labor. Contractions during pregnancy are called *Braxton-Hicks contractions.* Not all women feel them, and it doesn't matter if you don't. As labor starts, the contractions of the uterus become longer and stronger. And, unlike Braxton-Hicks contractions, they come at regular intervals. Some women first notice their labor pains when they are coming at perhaps five-minute intervals. The contractions may remain at this level throughout labor. Others become aware labor has started when they are having two or three contractions an hour. Then, as labor progresses, they find the contractions get closer together until they are two minutes apart.

Before you go to the hospital or before you call the doctor or midwife, just follow your normal routine as much as you can. *"I ate a light lunch and kept busy around the house until the middle of the afternoon. By that time I could no longer focus on anything except what was happening in my body."*

"Barry and I settled down to watch videos. I was leaning on a huge pile of sofa cushions. Within about an hour, things seemed to go up a notch. The contractions became stronger, more intense, longer and regular. During each one, I buried my head in the pillows and groaned to myself. When the contraction was over, I went back to watching the video."

It often happens that as soon as you get to the hospital or phone for the midwife to come to your home, contractions stop. Even though you were convinced you were in strong labor, the contractions just disappear: *"I didn't realize my contractions could just stop for no apparent reason."*

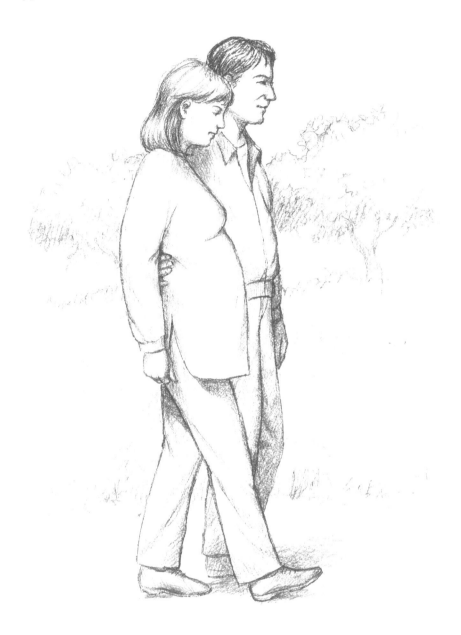

"On Monday, I started to get really strong contractions, every 5 to 6 minutes, for about two hours. So I called my doctor's office. As soon as I got to the office, everything stopped. I went home and had a good sleep."

Eating and Drinking during Labor

For many years, health providers told women they should not eat or drink anything besides water once they were in labor. Hospitals were strict about this. The fear was that if the mother needed to have a Cesarean-section delivery because something went wrong during labor, the food in her stomach, or the acid used to digest it, might pass into her lungs while she was unconscious under a general anesthetic. Now we know the amount of acid in your stomach does not decrease when you don't eat, it increases.

Despite this, some hospitals still don't allow women in labor to eat. Instead, they give them antacids every four hours to neutralize the acid in their stomachs. But antacids don't neutralize stomach acid nearly as well as small amounts of food taken at regular intervals.

You may hear it said that you should not eat in labor because food will take a long time to digest. The thing that really slows down digestion in labor is taking Demerol® for pain relief. It's safer to have light snacks in labor and not have Demerol than to have Demerol and go hungry. Many doctors and midwives now feel that telling a woman she can't eat in labor is a mistake.

The arguments for eating in labor are:

- Women in labor are engaged in hard physical work. They need food for energy, or they can become exhausted. Eating during labor can make contractions and the whole birth process more efficient.

- When you have not eaten for a long time, you feel weak, bad-tempered and unable to cope. The same principle applies to women in labor.

- Research carried out in the United States has shown that women who are allowed to eat during labor have fewer forceps and ventouse (vacuum) births and fewer Cesareans. They feel happier about their labors and have healthier babies.

Food is a major part of our enjoyment of life. It is also essential to keep us alive. Even the great religions of the world that dictate that people should fast at certain times make an exception for pregnant women!

Decide how you feel about eating in labor. Talk it over with your doctor or midwife. See if you can come to an agreement.

Going from your home to the hospital, or deciding that you're really in labor by asking the midwife to come to you, is a big step. If you are very excited about your labor, very anxious and "uptight," your body will respond by making lots of adrenaline. That's the hormone of "fright and flight." Adrenaline works against the oxytocin that is making your womb contract. So the contractions stop. This is a very clever device on nature's part. Nature presumes that if you are frightened, you and your baby must be in danger. It makes sense to have a way of stopping labor until you are no longer frightened and feel safe enough to give birth to your baby. Once you have settled into your room at the hospital or welcomed the midwife into your house, you will start to relax and feel more secure. Soon contractions will get going again and your labor will continue.

What contractions are like

Most of the time, when women have normal labors without medical intervention, the pain of labor is manageable. It really helps to have people with you who are well known to you, who understand you and can respond to your needs. Contractions are like waves. The waves build up slowly, gaining in strength all the time. Then they reach a crest when they crash down and race towards the shore, losing their power and finally trickling away into nothing on the beach. When the wave is finished, there is a slight pause before the next one begins. *"It's bearable because it's not continuous pain. You get a break in between."*

Contractions start as small waves that become bigger and stronger as labor progresses. Most of the time, the woman has time to adjust herself to the increasing strength of her labor. *"It doesn't come suddenly. It builds up. If you can deal with it mentally and not get too tense, then you can get through the later stages. You can learn as you go along how to cope."*

"You get used to it. Your body helps you."

Contractions in the first part of labor can be felt in various parts of the body. But they're rarely felt at the front where your tummy is.

"I felt the contractions in my back. They were really intense and not where I thought I would feel them."

"The contractions were in my groin. It really hurt."

"The contractions were down in my bottom, very low."

When the baby is being pushed out into the world during the second part of labor, the contractions feel very different. *"The contractions were like passing a watermelon. A very, very hard object! I remember thinking that while I was pushing."*

Despite the pain of contractions, women can still find labor an exciting event: *"The entire time, there's excitement underneath."*

How labor progresses

In the early part of labor, women often feel restless. They try all kinds of ways to make themselves more comfortable. *"It was getting harder to cope. I was very restless. I kept going to the bathroom, trying to throw up. I rocked back and forth during contractions."*

No one can say how long a first labor will last. It could take a couple of hours or a couple of days. *"It was short and really intense. There wasn't time to think about it or get my act together. It was just happening. The contractions came like a tidal wave."*

"My labor was long, a 45-hour marathon. I had lots of time to think. I even baked a pie during the first stage! What I mainly remember is being really tired because I didn't sleep for two nights."

The second time around, labor may be shorter than it was the first time—but there's no guarantee: *"My second labor was twice as long as my first. It lasted 18 hours. But until the very last part, I think it was easier than my first."*

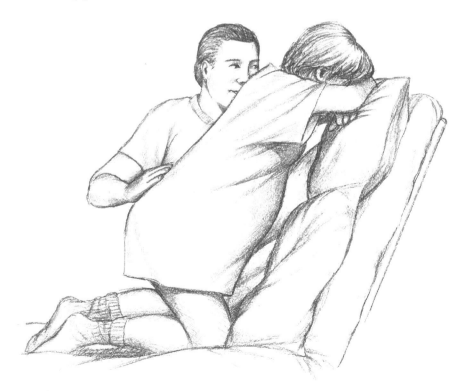

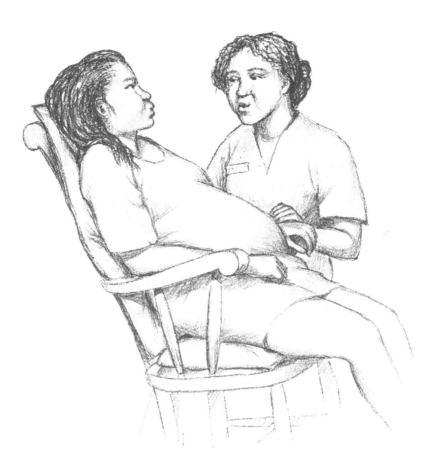

Many women find they are not aware of time passing. They don't notice the hours slip by. *"I lost all sense of time from one morning to the next. I don't remember much about some of the labor."*

At the end of the first stage, contractions often come fast and furious and are intense and painful. Women often feel they can't cope any longer. This part of labor is sometimes called *transition: "I kept saying, 'I want to go home! I want to go home!' I'd had enough."*

"When I look back on it, I think I had a pretty positive labor except for the last half-hour before I started pushing. This was the only point when I said, 'Just give me an epidural. I can't take any more.'"

"My transition seemed long. I flailed around, yelling at the nurses, 'Tell me what to do! I can't think any more!'"

Your uterus is working extra-hard during this part of labor to open your cervix fully to let your baby come through and be born. Your labor-support person and nurse-midwife are probably working hard also. They will be doing all they can to make you feel better. While you are completely involved in contractions, transition may be a very anxious time for your support person. If this person is your partner, he may be feeling fairly helpless. He will be wondering what he can possibly do to help you more. And he may worry that what is happening may not be normal, and that you and the baby might be in danger. He may also have to cope with a very bad temper on your part. Women have been known to verbally abuse their partners at this point in labor!

It can be hard to stay positive while you are going through transition. You may be feeling nauseated and shivery and bad-tempered. But all those things are signs the first stage of labor is almost over! You're almost done! After transition comes the second stage of labor, when your womb starts to push your baby out into the world.

Giving birth

Once your doctor or midwife tells you the second stage of labor has started, you probably will feel much more hopeful again and ready to push. In the first stage of labor, you may have felt you were simply enduring the contractions. But in the second stage, you can push actively. This can be very satisfying.

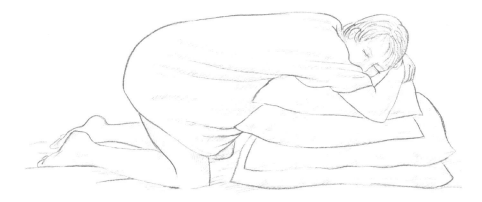

Transition

At the end of the first stage of labor, when the cervix is almost fully open, a range of symptoms appear. These mark the transition between the first and second stages of labor. Symptoms include:

- Shaking
- Suddenly feeling very cold
- Icy feet
- Hiccuping
- Burping
- Feeling nauseated or throwing up
- Feeling weepy and helpless and wanting to give up
- Feeling very angry with everyone, including the baby, because labor hurts so much
- Being bad-tempered and abusive

The fact is, labor is hard work at this point. Women often feel they can't cope much longer. But they won't have to because it's almost time to push! They need lots and lots of encouragement now. You need to be reassured that what you are feeling means you're almost ready to push your baby out into the world and hold him for the first time.

Don't worry—very few women have *all* the symptoms outlined above. Some women have none of them!

After transition, it is common for contractions to stop completely for ten or twenty minutes. This gives the mother time to rest and renew her energy for pushing. Nature does not lack compassion!

Feeling that you want to push before the cervix is fully open

You may feel you want to push, but your doctor or midwife tells you your cervix is not open far enough to let the baby come through. Try the following strategies to control the pushing urge:

- Kneel on the bed or on the floor with your face on the mattress and your bottom in the air. This position will reduce the pushing sensation.
- Try panting—three short pants and one long exhalation. Say to yourself: "I . . . will . . . not . . . push."
- Have your labor-support person push up on your tail bone with strong, steady pressure.

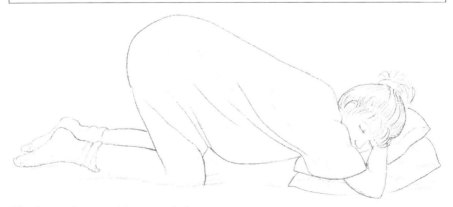

The knee-chest position can help a woman cope with an early urge to push.

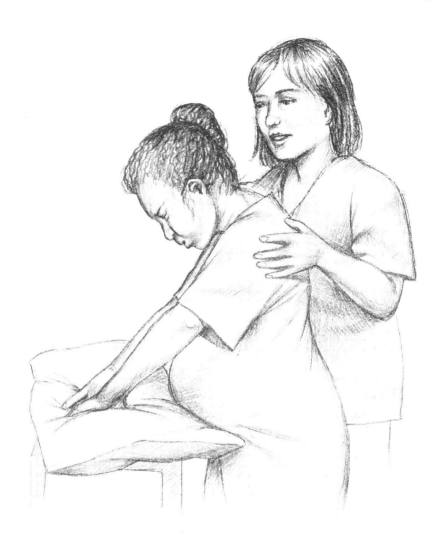

"I just wanted to push. When you get that feeling, the pain seems to disappear. It changes."

"Pushing felt completely instinctive—as if some kind of animal energy was taking over in me."

The second stage can also be intense and frightening. The painful contractions of transition are gone. But second stage brings other powerful pressures as you work to push the baby out. These sensations can be much stronger than those of the first stage and women use powerful words to describe how they felt.

"The baby's head moving down was very frightening. I really felt like I would split open."

"I had an awful stinging sensation when the head was being born. I remember thinking, 'I can't deliver this baby.' It was very painful, and it was frightening to push and feel the pain again."

Some women don't get an urge to push but still try to push or are told to push. Their bodies aren't telling them to push. This can make labor distressing and extremely hard work. *"Labor itself was only five hours. But my contractions had turned off by the second stage. I had two hours of hell trying to push the baby out with no urge to push."*

If you don't use any pain-relief drugs during labor, your uterus will have more than enough power to get your baby born without you pushing at all. If you don't want to push, tell your doctor or midwife and listen to what your body is saying to you. Perhaps it would be helpful to try another position. Perhaps it would be best just to breathe deeply, following your breath right down between your legs in order to help your baby be born. Some childbirth educators feel it's better for women not to push during second stage. Then birth can be very gentle for them and their babies.

Labor is often noisy. And second stage is the noisiest. But the grunts the woman makes are helpful to her. They are part of the huge effort of giving birth. They also give important clues to the doctor or midwife about what is happening. *"I made a lot of noise in second stage."*

"My doctor used the noises I was making to know where I was [in labor]. She didn't examine me. She was terrific."

"I began to get the urge to push. I was aware of making a lot of noise at this point. But it was a wonderful way to work through the intense pressure I felt."

Very fast labors

Sometimes women find they are in second-stage labor almost before they have realized they are in labor at all! Babies who are born suddenly at home or on the way to the hospital come very easily most of the time. In the following story, the mother crouched with her chest on the floor and her bottom in the air to try and give her husband time to get her to the hospital. *"It was still about a half-hour's drive to the hospital and my waters broke. I wanted to push when we were about halfway there. I was on my hands and knees on the back seat of the car with my rear in the air, trying not to push. We got to the hospital and the nurse said to me, 'What stage are you in?' At this point I was on the floor with my backside in the air, saying, 'I want to push!' And she said, 'Don't be silly. Come into this room and give me a urine sample.' I thought, 'You've got to be kidding! I'm having a baby!' But when she checked me she said I could push because the head was there. So I got up and squatted and just pushed and he was out! He was a 9 lb., 14 oz. baby. It was a very pleasurable experience."*

The moment of birth

Some women choose to lift their babies out of their bodies themselves, and take them right into their arms for the first cuddle. *"The baby's head eased out with the next contraction. It was such a relief to see this little dark head between my legs. We had to wait a couple of minutes for*

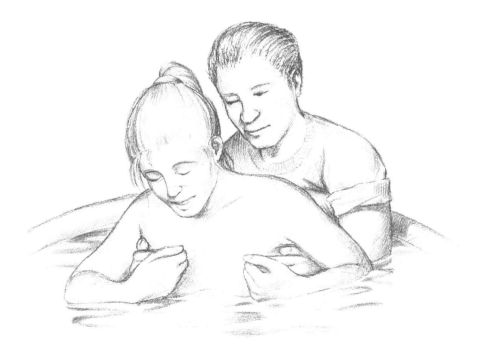

the next contraction before the rest of her body was born. As she came out, I put my hands down and lifted her onto me."

For other women, the moment of birth is equally joyous, but different, because they are having a Cesarean section: *"I heard a gush as my waters broke and I felt a tugging sensation inside me. Then the doctor called out: 'It's really big, it's a really big boy!' She lifted him above the screen so I could see him. Then he was placed face-down on my chest. He started to suck right away. It was the best moment of my life."*

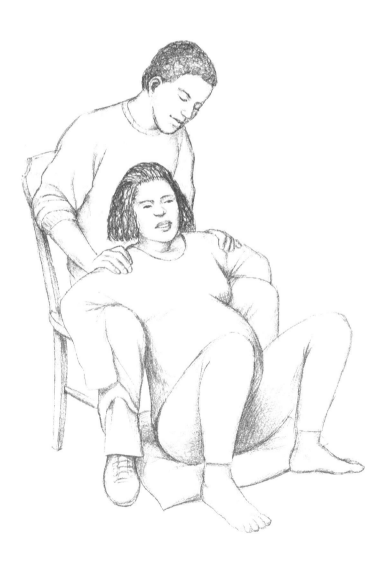

Twin births are different in other ways. *"Suddenly the room was full of people. It seems like the whole world wants to see twins being born! My legs were in stirrups because the first baby was breech and I was having forceps. The doctor gave me a local anesthetic because of the forceps. And then there was all this pushing and pulling. I was pushing and he was pulling. I felt a twang when the baby's legs came out. The doctor held her up for a moment so we could see her. Then she was whisked away to be checked. I wanted to push again and Joshua arrived face-up. The doctor placed him on my tummy. He looked exactly like my other two boys. Then they gave me Anna. There I was, with my legs still in the air and my arms full of babies!"*

The moment of birth is not always the big event the woman has been looking forward to. Some painkilling drugs can make women feel so doped that they hardly realize they have given birth. Or sometimes the baby may need special care and be taken to the neonatal intensive care unit (NICU). When this happens, some mothers feel they have been denied something very important. *"My husband held him, which I liked. But my memories are so vague . . . I feel really sad that I can't remember much about it."*

"I wasn't allowed to hold the baby. The nurse took him away and I didn't see him again for an hour. It felt strange when he was brought to me—like he wasn't really mine."

Some women are just too exhausted to take charge of the baby right away. *"I was very tired and they said, 'We'll take him to the nursery and give him some milk.' I said, 'Fine.' I wanted to go to sleep. I was wrung out."*

The baby may not look like what you were expecting. Some babies are purple when they are born. Some look grey and lifeless, which is frightening. In a very short time, they turn pink and look very different. *"He cried and I knew he was alive. He looked like a gray lump of clay, and they gave him some oxygen. Then he cried again and turned pink. Then they wrapped him up in a green sheet. I asked if I could pick him up. I haven't really put him down since."*

Labor often involves harder work than you have ever done before. You feel the strongest physical sensations you have ever known. The moment of birth, too, can be charged with intense emotion. *"I said, 'Oh! Oh! It's a boy! It's a boy!' and I started crying and Jake started crying.'"*

The birth of the baby helps put the events of labor into perspective.

"Whatever you go through, once you see the baby at the end, you forget it. At least I did!"

"I couldn't believe I'd had a baby and everything was OK."

Some women feel so empowered by labor, so strong and confident, that they are ready to do it all over again! They have a feeling of immense pride in what they have achieved.

"It had been a long labor and I was exhausted. But I had a tremendous feeling of achievement. I had succeeded in giving birth!"

"I'd have another baby tomorrow! It's just the most amazing thing."

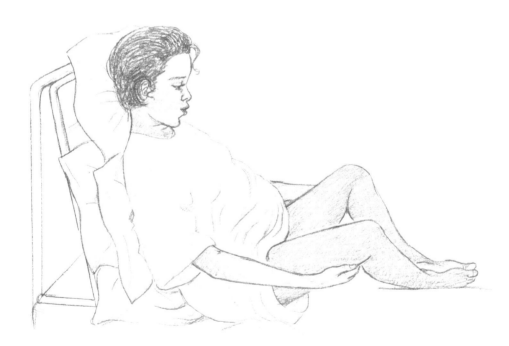

Tips from Women Who Have Given Birth

Women who have just had babies themselves are often the best source of good advice on how to prepare for labor and how to cope when it happens:

"It's really important to be well prepared so you understand what's going on. Go to classes and read a lot."

"I think you need to know all your options for pain relief beforehand. At the time, you can't think about what's being offered. It's better to have looked into it at the beginning of pregnancy."

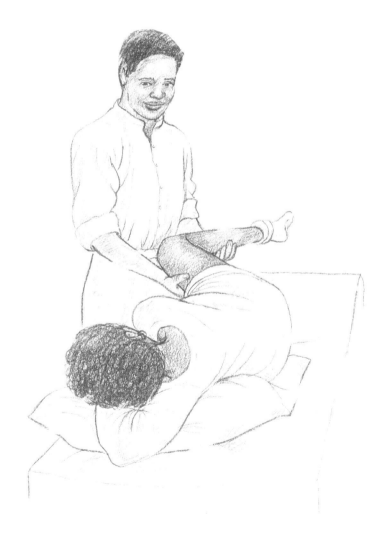

Third Stage of Labor

The third stage of labor is when contractions push the placenta or afterbirth out of the uterus. These contractions are not likely to be painful. Third-stage labor can happen in two ways.

"Managed" third stage

- As your baby's shoulders are being born, you are given a shot in your thigh of a drug called *syntometrine*
- As soon as your baby is born, his umbilical cord is clamped in two places and cut in between. He will no longer be attached to you.
- The syntometrine makes your uterus contract strongly to force out the placenta.
- The midwife pulls on the cord, which is still attached to the placenta inside you, to help out the placenta
- The placenta is delivered within 5 to 7 minutes of the birth of your baby.

"Natural" third stage

- When your baby is born, his umbilical cord is not clamped.
- You put your baby to the breast and encourage him to suckle. This stimulates your body to produce more oxytocin to make your uterus contract and push out the placenta.
- The midwife or nurse waits and observes.
- The time from the birth of your baby to the delivery of the placenta could be anywhere from ten minutes to 1-1/2 hours.

The Placenta and Afterbirth

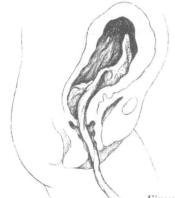

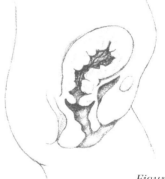

Figure 1   *Figure 2*

The placenta or afterbirth comes away from the wall of the uterus after the baby has been born. It drops into the lower part of the womb. From there it is pushed out by the mother or helped out by the midwife (figure 1). Then the womb contracts (figure 2).

Natural Third Stage

Benefits

Nature is allowed to take its course.

When your baby is born, he has two sources of oxygen. He is still receiving oxygen from you through his umbilical cord because it hasn't been clamped. And he is starting to breathe for himself. If he has amniotic fluid in his lungs or has any trouble breathing, the doctor or midwife has plenty of time to extract the fluid and help him start to breathe on his own.

Your baby gets exactly the amount of blood nature intended him to have. The umbilical cord will pulse for up to ten minutes after his birth.

Problems

You can only have a natural third stage if you have had a natural labor. You *cannot* use pain-relief drugs, an epidural, or an IV drip to stimulate contractions. You have to have been upright and mobile for most of your labor.

Third stage may take a long time.

You may lose more blood than if you had had syntometrine.

Managed Third Stage

Benefits

Third stage is over very quickly.

Women are at risk of bleeding heavily in the third stage of labor. The injection you are given controls bleeding. At the moment, research suggests that women who have the injection bleed less than women who don't.

Problems

Because your baby's umbilical cord is clamped as soon as he is born, he is no longer getting oxygen from you. He must breathe on his own right away. If he has amniotic fluid in his lungs or has any problem breathing right away, it can be a real emergency.

Clamping the cord means blood is left in the cord that would normally have passed to the baby.

If the cord isn't clamped, blood rushes along it like a tidal wave when the syntometrine makes your uterus contract. This sudden rush of blood may not be a problem for a healthy baby. But it could be hard on a baby who is not strong.

Syntometrine closes the cervix quickly. If for some reason the placenta isn't born within seven minutes, it will be trapped inside the womb. You will need to have it taken out in an operating room. This is called "a retained placenta." Three percent to 5% of women have this problem.

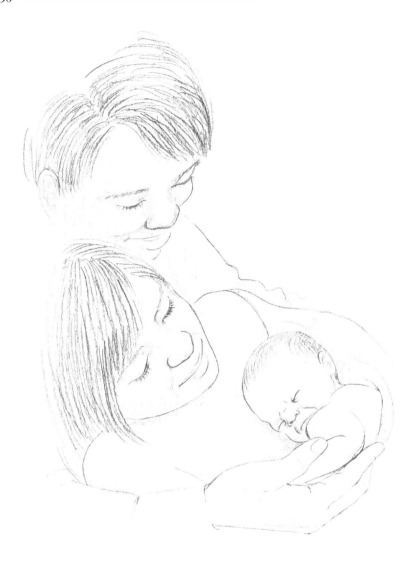

"If you're worried about something, ask and they will tell you."

"Relax and let nature take its course. As long as you have people there to help who know what's going on, there's nothing to worry about."

"Your body tells you a lot of what to do."

"Remember that it's only one day in your life and the baby's."

And finally, you have to recognize that:

"Nothing can totally prepare you!"

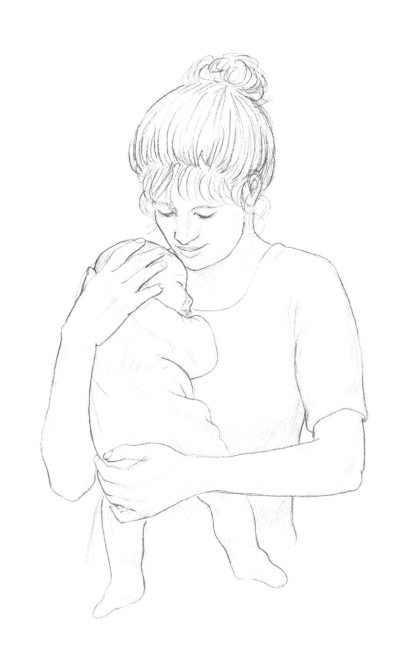

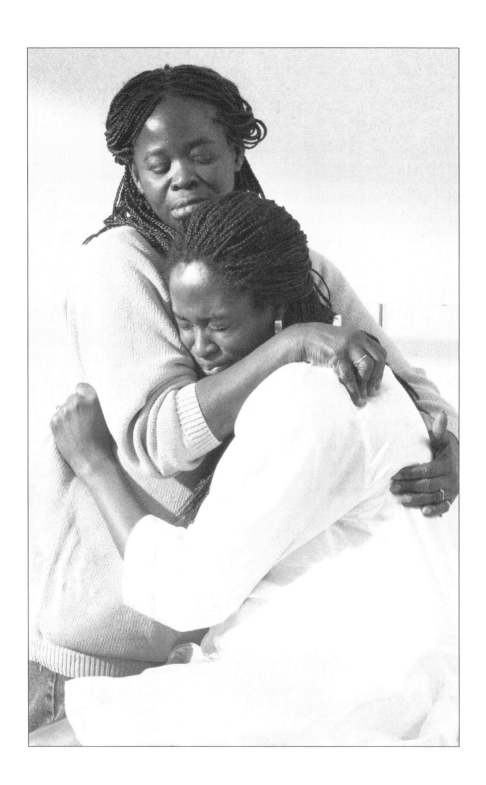

CHAPTER 5
Coping with Pain in Labor

What about Pain?

Most pregnant women are anxious about pain in labor. What will it be like? How bad will it be? Will they be able to cope? Movies show us labors that look long, painful and often dangerous. Women who have given birth sometimes tell horror stories about their labors. (Many of these stories become more dramatic in the retelling.) When pregnant women go to their prenatal classes, they find that their teacher spends a lot of time talking about pain in labor. She suggests practical ways of coping. She may also discuss drugs and procedures for pain relief. Some women become frightened thinking about pain in labor. This can spoil the last months of their pregnancies:

"I know my body can do it but I'm scared. They say if you're scared, your body tenses and then you feel more pain. It becomes a vicious cycle. I'm scared of getting into that and not being able to get out again. I try not to think about [what will happen] when I go into labor. The more I think about it, the more scared I am."

"I try not to listen to people's horror stories. There is so much fear around. It's hard to break through that and remain confident."

"I buy all the baby magazines. When I was about three months pregnant, there was one article called Everything You Need to Know about Stitches. *It went into really graphic detail about all the things that could go wrong. I was in tears because I was so worried about labor."*

Coping with Back Labor

Sometimes your baby lies with his back against your back. Your doctor calls this *a posterior position.* When the baby is in this position, you may have a backache during your labor. The backache comes not just with the contractions, but between them, too. This makes it harder for you to rest, relax and prepare for the next contraction.

A number of things might help:

- Try getting down on all fours during contractions so your baby drops away from your spine. This helps relieve the pressure on your back.

- Your labor-support person or nurse can wrap a hot-water bottle in a towel and place it in the small of your back. You may also find something very cold helps the ache, such as an ice-cold water bottle wrapped in a towel.

- Firm pressure or massage to the lower part of your back may help. Your labor coach can try placing the heel of his hand firmly against your tailbone. Then have him press up or move his hand in small, firm circles. If you don't like this, say so!

- Help your baby move around by making as much room in your pelvis as you can. Keep moving. Try squatting for a while. Squatting opens the pelvis as much as possible. Rock your hips forward and back (like doing the "bump"), or move them in circles and from side to side.

You can do so much to help yourself in labor! Women often cope with pain much better than they think they can. Scary old-wives' tales always focus on the hard parts of labor instead of on the joyful and exciting parts. It would be more helpful to the little girls who will one day be mothers if adults gave them a more balanced picture of labor.

How the Pain Helps

The first thing to say about pain in labor is that some women do not have any. These women may be few in number. But a great many other women feel that the pain of labor is no big deal. These women found that labor was very much within the range of what they had felt before in their daily lives:

"I didn't feel any pain. I wouldn't call it pain at all. I'm not saying it felt good. It wasn't comfortable. I was very aware that it was all happening. But it wasn't painful. And I was very much alert and arguing!"

"I felt intense period pains. They weren't pleasant, but I didn't feel pain in any frightening way."

In fact, not feeling pain in labor can be a problem. Many women expect that part of the transition to motherhood involves going through a painful labor.

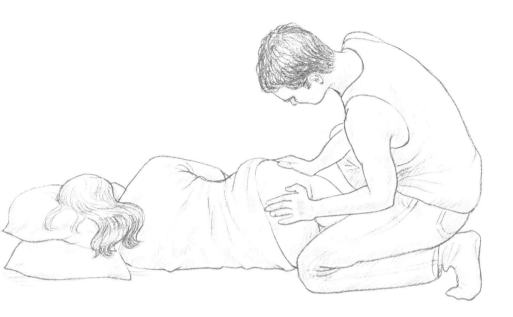

Firm pressure or massage to the tailbone
may help ease back-labor pain.

Women sometimes feel that the pain of labor is an important test of their commitment to the baby:

"I did feel contractions, but they weren't intense. I really miss that. I think I should have had that. Next time, I'm looking forward to having some pain!"

"More and more I feel the pain of labor is a good thing. Not that I enjoyed it—well, I did in some ways. For me, a pain-free labor isn't what I'm after—no sense of achievement."

It seems unlikely that the pain of labor should be beyond what most women can bear. Nature intends the pain to serve some very useful purposes. The first painful contractions tell the mother that she is in labor. If mothers felt nothing at all, babies would be born in some very awkward places! The slow increase in strength of contractions gives the mother a sign of how far along in labor she is. Thus, as the time comes for her baby to be born, she can summon help and go to a safe place to give birth.

Helping Yourself Cope with Pain

Finding Comfort

Most of all, you want to get *comfortable!* Whether you are having your baby at home or in a hospital, move around all the time. Try new positions to see which is best for you. Chances are, what makes you feel best will also make it easier for your baby to be born.

Nearly all women find that being upright in labor helps them cope with the pain better. The bones of your pelvis can open wider if you are upright than if you are sitting on your tailbone. Gravity also helps your baby move down through your pelvis. When the uterus contracts, it moves forward. You may find it feels better to lean forward yourself. This way, you help the uterus perform its job.

You can try all sorts of positions. The only guide is what works best for you. As you go through labor, you may want to change your position many times.

- Stand and lean forward onto a table, the back of a chair, a bed or your labor-support person.

- Kneel, lean onto the seat of a chair, or onto your labor-support person's knees if he is sitting. Or try leaning onto a bean bag or a pile of pillows.

- Get down on all fours with your head dropped down.

- Sit "cowboy style" astride a chair. Lean onto a pillow placed across the back of the chair.

- Lie on your left side with a pillow between your legs if you are very tired.

- Squat and support yourself by leaning forward onto your hands. Or hold onto your partner's knees while he is sitting.

- Sit on the toilet. Get your partner to kneel in front of the toilet. Then lean forward and rest your head on your partner's shoulder.

You will find many of these positions more helpful if you combine them with rocking your hips forward and backward or around in circles. Rocking has been a form of comfort since ancient times. You will find it soothing. It also helps your baby explore your pelvis and find the best way through.

Make Noise

Feel free to make noise! Don't think you shouldn't, or that it's not the right thing to do. Don't worry that someone might think you are a nuisance or a wimp. Making noise is an effective form of pain relief. Look at the way small children react when they're hurt! Labor is often a noisy time. If it helps to groan, shout or make funny grunting noises, then do so.

Massage

When you hit yourself against something, your first instinct is to rub the spot that was hurt. Rubbing makes the body release natural pain-killing hormones called endorphins. Massage is just one form of rubbing.

Many women find it helpful to have the lower part of their back massaged during labor. Some like a lot of pressure applied to their tailbone. This can reduce the pain or ache of labor like magic! Some don't want to be touched at all during contractions and prefer not to be disturbed. Some women like to be massaged between contractions to help them relax.

continued

Helping Yourself Cope with Pain

Massage, continued

Tell your labor-support person or midwife where you want to be massaged and when. Tell them what is helpful and what is not. Massage may be nicer if your support person uses an oil that is scent-free on his hands. Oil can prevent chafing when he rubs your skin.

Breathing

Women breathe in all sorts of different ways during labor. Some take long, slow breaths to carry them through the contractions. Some lift their breathing over their contractions, taking small, shallow breaths. Some breathe in steps, taking a small breath in, then another, and then a small breath out and another.

Just keep your breathing even and don't get panicky. You don't want to start gasping and end up feeling dizzy, sick and tingly. It can help to focus on the out breath. (Your body is programmed to breathe in.) But sometimes the out breath can be held back. So think "out" when breathing and let your tension flow away as you breathe out.

Using Water

Most of us find that a bath or shower helps us relax when we are stressed. Water soothes aching muscles. The same is true in labor. Lying immersed in warm water helps many women relax and cope well with their contractions. If the water is deep enough, you will be able to use different positions to increase your comfort. If you don't have access to a birthing pool or bath, try taking a shower during labor instead.

Relaxation

All the things described above will help you relax. If you can relax, you will conserve your energy and ensure a good supply of oxygen to your baby. (Don't forget: Your baby is also going through labor!) It also helps if you get along well with your nurse or midwife. Then you feel free to ask her questions, which can also help you relax. Your labor-support person can use his own knowledge of what relaxes you to help you. If you go to prenatal classes, your teacher will help you learn to notice when you are getting tense and how to let go of your tension.

We respond to pain through instinct. If you bang your head on a cupboard door, you may rub your head. Rubbing helps your body make endorphins, a natural pain-killing hormone. If your stomach aches, you may lie down and curl up with a hot-water bottle. Warmth and being in a certain position can provide comfort. Pain tells us how to help ourselves when we've been injured. In labor, there is no injury. But pain helps teach a woman how to give birth. She is led by it to change her position to increase her comfort. By moving around and using different positions, she also helps her baby's head press down firmly all around the cervix. This helps the cervix open evenly. Later in labor, her changes in position can shift the baby one way and then the other. This helps him to find the best way down through her pelvis.

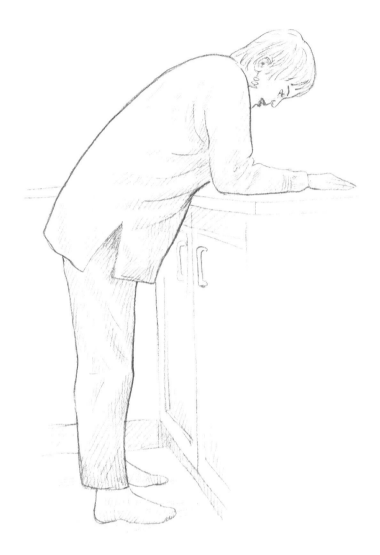

Keeping active

Most women feel restless at the start of labor and for the first few hours. They keep moving. Besides being nervous, women learn that moving around and being upright makes them feel better:

"I sat down a few times, but that didn't feel right. I just wanted to be standing up. I paced around the room."

"I was encouraged to walk around. In fact, I was sent back up to the ward to walk around rather than staying in delivery."

"I was in a rocking chair most of the night. I asked for a rocking chair, and it was really good."

Nature is full of rhythm—the beating of the heart, the pattern of sleeping and waking, a woman's monthly cycle. The way contractions rise to a climax and then subside is also rhythmical. Women often use rhythm to help them cope: *"There was only a small space in the delivery room to walk around in. I did sort of a rhythmic pacing up and down, trying to relax and focus."*

"What made pain worse was being still at any stage. What made the pain better was leaning forward, swaying my hips from side to side and then around and around."

Later on, when labor has progressed and contractions are stronger, women move around less. But still they do not often choose to sit or lie down:

"I couldn't walk or even stand up—I had to kneel, it was so painful."

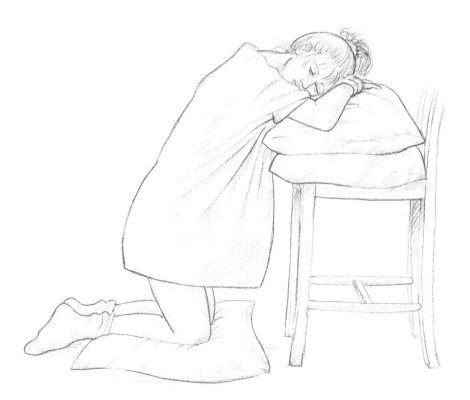

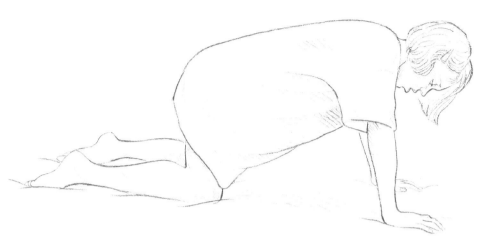

"As the contractions got a little stronger, I went to my hands and knees. It helped ease the weight on my back."

"I just didn't want to lie down on the bed. It made the contractions much harder to cope with."

Touch during labor

It really helps to have the freedom to move around during labor. You need to choose the positions that make you feel best. The support you receive from your labor coach and nurse or midwife can also make a big difference. Their positive words are vital. But even more important can be the way in which they touch and hold you.

A back rub or massage during labor helps because the pressure feels good. The physical contact with someone who cares for you and is trying hard to help you is also an excellent form of pain relief. Women need to be loved during labor!

"I was getting pain in the lower spine. Just pressure there or rubbing seemed to take the edge off."

"What really helped me was massage—I wanted more, harder, harder! It was wonderful. I suppose it added pressure. But it took away a lot of the pain at the same time. It was wonderful."

"When I was having contractions, I needed to hold somebody's hand. I was offered medication. But I grabbed somebody's hand instead. That really got me through it."

If the baby is being born by Cesarean section, the woman still needs to have physical contact with someone who is caring for *her: "During the operation, he was just stroking my head, which made me feel better."*

Using water

It is well known that warm water soothes the pain of labor. More and more hospitals are installing showers or tubs. Many doctors and midwives encourage women to take a bath during the first stage of labor.

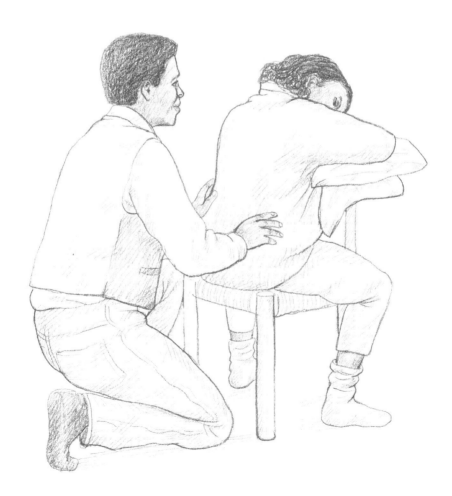

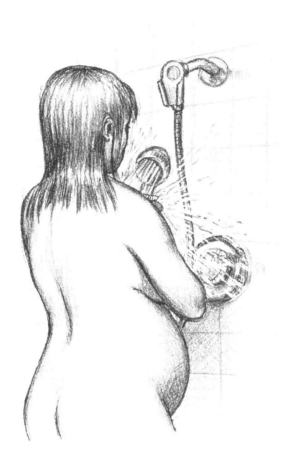

Some are even prepared to help women give birth in the water. If the mother labors at home, she is free to use her own bath or shower as she pleases. Some women describe how their pain almost disappeared, as if by magic, once they got into the water:

"The pool looked so good to me. I got in when I was 6cm dilated. It was great—just like I'd imagined. I could relax completely between contractions. I no longer waited in dread for the next one. Jason rubbed the small of my back. The effect, along with the warm water, was just wonderful."

"I had to be in the shower. I had to have really hot water pounding down on my back."

Just as for other forms of pain relief in labor, though, what suits one woman will not suit another. Each woman is unique in the way in which her body responds to pain and in the things she finds helpful. For some women, getting into a pool is not soothing at all:

"I was helpless in the bathtub. It wasn't a big round bathtub, just a normal, long, thin tub. I had a pretty intense contraction as I got in. I kept thinking, 'I wish I could get out.' I wanted to be standing up. I didn't feel very secure in the tub."

If you can use a bathtub or a birthing pool during labor, and the thought appeals to you, give it a try. If you don't think the water is helpful, that's OK. Just get out and try something else. You've lost nothing by giving it a try.

Breathing and relaxation

Prenatal classes often spend a lot of time helping women understand their breathing patterns. Women can learn how to use their breathing to cope with pain in labor. Learning to relax is also a big part of such classes. But can women put into practice what they have learned? Breathing techniques do seem to be helpful:

"What made it better for me was the breathing drills. They really work. You don't think they will, but they do. You've got to focus. If you let your mind wander, you've lost it. You've got to focus totally on the breathing you're doing."

"For me, breathing helped with the contractions. Blowing out during the contraction—that really helped. It helped me so much that I was 8cm dilated when I got to the hospital."

It may not be easy to relax during labor. But women who try to relax find that it makes a big difference: *"It's very hard to relax, you know. You feel your tummy get hard and the rest of you seems to clench up. You even clench your fists and grind your teeth. You have to force yourself to relax and calm down. It does help when you relax. It really does."*

"I tried to relax during the contractions. I turned on my portable CD player with earphones. We'd taped my favorite songs a few weeks before. I listened to them over and over. That helped me relax."

Alternative Forms of Pain Relief

For an alternative form of pain relief, you could try one of these therapies:

Acupuncture
Aromatherapy
Homoeopathy
Hypnotherapy
Reflexology

These therapies may help with problems in pregnancy and after the baby is born. They can also be used to help a woman cope with pain in labor.

Some doctors or nurses are trained in one or more of these therapies. They may offer it to women in their care. Such therapists take a holistic approach to care. They treat people as a whole. They look at their whole lives and moods as much as at their bodily symptoms.

Research into most of these therapies is still in its infancy. At present, there is no strong evidence that most of them are safe and effective. But more and more research is being carried out. And people who practice these therapies are adopting codes of conduct similar to those of regular healthcare providers.

For more information about these therapies, you can:

• Talk to other women who have tried it.

• Get a list of registered or trained therapists.

• Contact a local therapist. Ask how much she charges for a consultation. Ask what kind of help you can expect.

• Talk to your doctor or midwife about the therapy that interests you. There may be a local healthcare provider who has some knowledge of it or who is trained as a therapist.

• Read books and magazine articles. Learn as much as you can.

These therapies can be used to treat morning sickness, varicose veins, hemorrhoids, headaches, heartburn and depression.

They can also be used to help with slow labors. They may help reduce pain in labor and control bleeding after labor. They can be tried with babies who cry a lot. And they may help babies who suffer from colic or who have been traumatized by their birth.

Many of the things you learned in prenatal classes, from reading books or from other women, will not be helpful on the big day. Think of breathing techniques, positions and the relaxation you practice as tools for labor. When the day comes, you will look through the tools you have collected and choose the ones that seem to work for you. The rest you set aside to use later, or perhaps not at all:

"Labor felt just like very strong period pains. Being touched made it worse. After all the massage we practiced, I didn't want to be touched at all! Using different positions, though, felt just right."

"My breathing went completely out the window. I thought I was doing the right thing, but the nurses said I wasn't. I was panting when I wasn't supposed to be. I think it was panic. I forgot all the things we'd learned except making noises. Shouting worked great!"

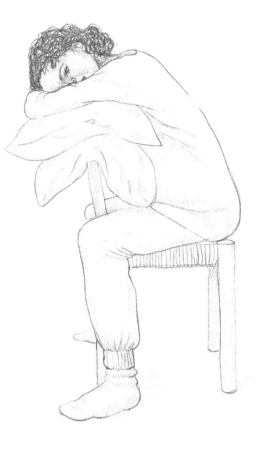

Medical Forms of Pain Relief

If you are having a home birth, you probably won't be offered drugs for pain in labor. Don't worry. Many women find that non-medical methods of pain relief work better for them than drugs. In the hospital, you can choose from all these options. You could also have an epidural. You have to decide whether the amount of help you will get from using drugs in labor is worth the trouble they can cause.

Pethidine (Demerol®)

Pethidine is a narcotic, like morphine. It is still widely used for pain relief in labor. But it is not used nearly as much as it was before epidurals came on the scene. Pethidine rarely gets rave reviews from women who have used it. Some women find it helps them rest and perhaps even grab a few hours' sleep during labor. But others find that the drowsiness pethidine causes doesn't carry them over the top of contractions. Pethidine also seems to make them feel completely out of control of what is happening to them.

"Pethidine didn't help me. I would wake up at the height of each con-traction. I couldn't cope with the pain at that point."

"I was tired, exhausted. They said, 'You need pethidine.' Why do they offer pethidine when you are losing control? It makes you lose control more."

Pethidine can sometimes knock out a woman so completely that she doesn't even know her baby has been born: *"Labor is just a blur to me. I couldn't tell you how Sophie was born."*

Some women will not consider having pethidine because they are afraid it might deprive them of the first moments of their babies' lives: *"The only thing I know is that I want to be conscious. I want to be there. Anything that's likely to cloud your mind, like pethidine, I would not want. It means a lot to me to be completely alert when I meet our baby."*

If you do decide to have pethidine in labor because you don't want an epidural, talk with your doctor or midwife about having a smaller dosage, perhaps 25mg or 50mg instead of 100mg. You can always have more pethidine if you want it. But once it's been given, you can't take it back if it turns out to have been too much.

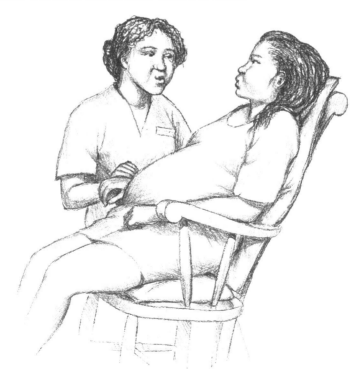

Methods of Pain Relief

Pethidine

The facts:

- Pethidine is a drug related to morphine. It tends to make you drowsy. It can also disorient you.
- It is given in a shot, often into your thigh or bottom.
- A standard dose is 100mg. But some doctors give less. A smaller dose is used if you are small or lightly built. Pethidine can be given more than once during labor.
- The doctor or nurse will not want you to have pethidine if she thinks you are within a few hours of giving birth. Pethidine crosses the placenta. It will affect your baby most strongly if it has been given shortly before you give birth. The danger is that it can depress your baby's breathing.

What's good about it:

- If a woman is tense during labor, contractions to open the cervix may not work as well. Pethidine may help a woman relax so her uterus can find its rhythm again.
- Some women will tell you pethidine was great for them because it allowed them to have a much-needed rest during labor. It has helped some women cope with the pain of contractions.

What's not so good about it:

- Pethidine doesn't only relieve pain. It also affects your breathing, which becomes slower and more shallow. Because it crosses the placenta, it may also affect the baby's breathing after he is born.
- Some women say that pethidine made them so drowsy that they were not even aware that their baby was being born. Missing the birth in this way can make a woman very unhappy about her labor afterwards.
- Some women find pethidine makes them too drowsy to know when a contraction is building. And it's not strong enough to carry them over the most painful part of the contraction. The result is that they tend to "wake up" at the most painful moment of each contraction.
- Pethidine can make mothers feel very sick. For this reason, it is often given with another drug to help control sickness.

Epidurals

Many women strongly favor epidurals. They feel an epidural allows a woman to regain control of her labor and of her dignity: *"I remember seeing this woman in labor on a video. She'd had an epidural and she was telling jokes. She had been screaming before then."*

An epidural can transform a labor that frightens a woman because of the pain involved into a time she remembers with pleasure: *"We sat there for two hours, and I only got to 1cm. I was really relieved when they said, 'Have an epidural.' I went to sleep for two hours and when I woke, I was 10cm. That's the way to do it! It was perfect. No suffering or pain at all."*

"*I was given a drip and had an epidural, which I thought was very good. I was with it when the baby was born. It was a positive thing. I wouldn't rule out having an epidural again."*

"*You don't know how you're going to react. I thought the labor was really hard. The epidural made it OK for me. I was so glad to have it."*

Although epidurals are replacing pethidine as the main form of pain relief for women in labor, they may not take away all the pain of the contractions. A few women find that their epidural doesn't work completely: "*I thought the epidural was frightening. It didn't work as high up as it should have. I could still feel contractions pushing up into my ribs."*

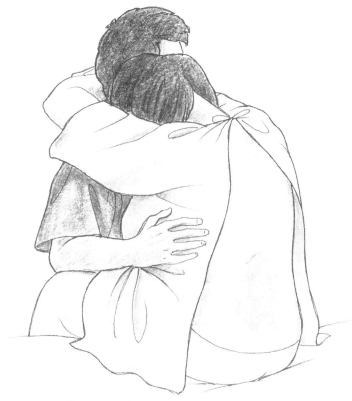

Getting into position for an epidural

Methods of Pain Relief

Epidurals

The facts:

- An epidural is set up by an anesthetist. If the hospital is busy, you may have to wait for an anesthetist. You can't have an epidural for a home birth.

- An epidural may cause your blood pressure to drop suddenly. So a doctor puts an IV drip into your arm. The drip means fluids can be given straight into your bloodstream to bring your blood pressure up again.

Next the anesthetist sprays the bottom of your back with a cold solution to numb the skin. He then puts a hollow needle into your back. He will feel carefully for the right spot just outside the protective layers that surround the spinal cord. A narrow tube called a *catheter* is threaded through the hollow needle. Then the needle is taken out. The catheter is taped over your shoulder.

The anesthetist injects a local pain-killing drug into the top end. This drug is often combined with a narcotic. You may feel a cold sensation in your back soon afterwards. You may then be asked to lie first on one side, then on the other to help the drug spread evenly.

After a few seconds, you start to lose feeling in your legs. Then the feeling of the contractions disappear. The epidural can be "topped up" by the doctor when you start to feel the contractions again.

- If you have an epidural during the early part of labor, you may have a tube (catheter) put into your bladder. This permits urine to drain freely into a bag attached to the tube. This has to be done because you will not be able to tell when you need to go to the toilet. A full bladder makes it harder for the baby to be born.

What's good about it:

- Epidurals give many women complete relief from labor pain.

- They can help a mother feel "in control" of her labor after feeling out of control because of intense contractions.

- If the mother needs stitches after giving birth, an epidural will provide pain relief while the stitching is done.

- If a Cesarean section is needed during labor, the epidural can be used for the operation. This means she can be awake when her baby is born. She won't need to have a general anesthetic.

What's not so good about it:

- A number of women, perhaps as many as 10% to 15%, do not get complete pain relief from an epidural. Some find they are numb on one side of the lower part of their body, but not on the other. Some women describe "windows of pain"—a small place on their stomach or back that doesn't seem to have been touched by the epidural. They can feel intense contractions in this one spot.

- An epidural may make some women feel out of control of their labor. With a tube in their back, an IV drip in their arm and perhaps a catheter in their bladder, they can't feel contractions at all. They must depend completely on healthcare providers to deliver their baby. They may not feel involved in the birth.

continued

Methods of Pain Relief

Epidural, continued

- When an epidural is used, it is harder to move around or change your position during labor. You probably won't be able to walk.

- If the epidural is still working in the second stage of labor when the baby is being born, the mother may not be able to push. There is a greater risk that she may need to have her baby delivered by forceps or suction. Both of these procedures carry their own risks for the baby.

- Sometimes the epidural needle pierces the cover that surrounds the spinal cord. This means the fluid that bathes the spinal cord leaks out slightly. This can give the mother a

horrible headache after the labor. The headache can be so bad that she is unable to care for her baby. A doctor may need to take some blood from her and inject it into her back to seal the hole made by the epidural needle.

- Some research suggests that some women may suffer from chronic low backache, shoulder ache and tingling of their arms and legs for weeks, months or years after having an epidural. It is not certain if these effects are due to the epidural itself or to the fact that the mother tends to remain in one position for her entire labor.

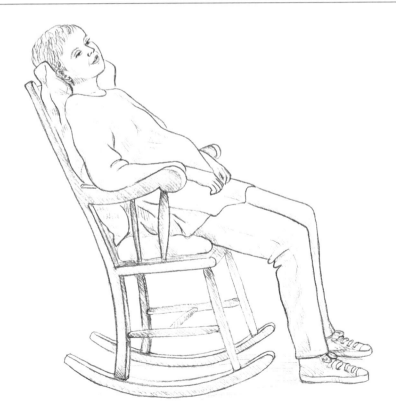

Methods of Pain Relief

Spinals

The facts:

A spinal anesthetic is an injection given into the lower part of the mother's back. It can only be given once, so the pain relief is short-term.

What's good about it:

• A spinal anesthetic can be given more quickly than an epidural. It starts to work right away. It is therefore very useful when the mother needs speedy pain relief. It can be used, for instance, when her baby needs to be born with the help of forceps or suction.

• A spinal can be used for a Cesarean section if the doctor is sure the operation will be without complications. A spinal wears off much more quickly than an epidural, so the mother has normal sensation again soon.

What's not so good about it:

• There is a greater risk of a sudden drop in the mother's blood pressure with a spinal than with an epidural.

• The injection pierces the cover around the spinal cord so that fluid may leak out. This can give the mother a severe headache after the birth of her baby.

• A spinal offers only short-term pain relief. It is of no use if labor is expected to be long.

An anesthetist sets up an epidural. He may bring another doctor to assist. Thus the delivery room may suddenly fill up with people. Some women dislike the loss of privacy that comes with an epidural: *"I didn't like the fact that I had to lie on the bed all the time, and there were a lot of doctors around. I would rather have had just my husband and a nurse."*

It may be a number of hours after the birth of her baby before a woman who has had an epidural completely regains the normal sensations in her legs and lower body. There can also be longer-term side-effects to cope with. There is research now to suggest that epidurals may cause some chronic back problems:

"I've had a lot of backaches since I gave birth to Paul. I'm not sure if it's because his head was in a funny position or if it's due to the epidural."

Preparing to Cope with Pain

While you are pregnant, you can think about how you're going to cope with pain in labor. You can consider which methods of pain relief, natural or medical, you would prefer. Some women decide about pain relief before labor starts: *"Before I actually went into labor, I felt strongly that I wasn't going to use any pain relief. I hate needles. I wanted to be fully aware of what was going on. I just felt I could manage without drugs. I wanted to show my boyfriend, too, because he thinks I'm a real wimp. In the end, just his massage got me through."*

But other women find that keeping an open mind might have been better: *"I had it written all across my chart: 'Does not want an epidural.' Did I feel silly! When I arrived at the hospital, I was screaming for one. I was awful to my husband, who was reminding me I didn't want an epidural. Now I think the best thing is to be open-minded."*

It may not be wise to have made all your decisions about which forms of pain relief to use in labor before the day arrives. But it does help to find out what your options might be in advance. If you are planning a home birth, what forms of pain relief can you use? Which forms of pain relief are used most often at the local hospitals? If you think you might want an epidural, you need to choose a hospital where you can get one 24 hours a day. If you feel you might not want to have a lot of drugs in labor, you might decide to have a home birth or give birth at a birthing center. Or you might choose a doctor or midwife who is known for helping women cope without drugs. You could also talk over your feelings about pain relief with your labor-support person. Being well prepared can make all the difference: *"You know that you can't imagine the pain beforehand. But if you prepare yourself by learning all you can, and you know what your choices are, you'll give yourself the best chance. Before I knew anything, I was so anxious. But now I feel prepared, and I have something to hold on to."*

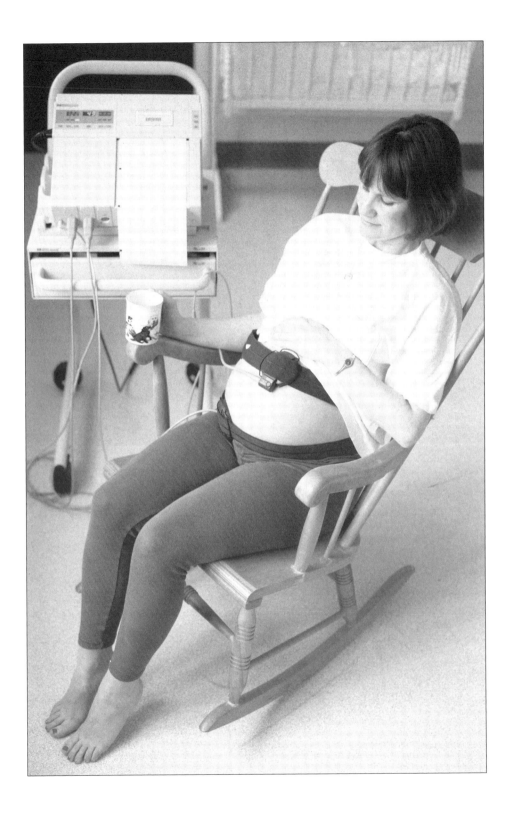

CHAPTER 6 *Interventions in Labor*

Pregnancy and labor are not illnesses. Having a baby is a normal part of a woman's life. Most women are perfectly able to give birth to their babies without any help at all. Most women in the developed parts of the world have enjoyed a good diet from birth. They have grown into healthy young women. In the United States and Canada, today's child-bearing women are the daughters of women who were fit and well nourished. It's likely they are the granddaughters of women who were also healthy. It is now safer than it ever was to give birth to a child. Hardly anyone knows of a woman who died while having a baby. And few women suffer the grief of giving birth to a stillborn child.

Having a baby in the United States or Canada today is very safe. We are, for the most part, healthy nations. We are able to drink clean water. The sewage systems work. Most of us are well-housed so that we don't suffer from the health problems that come with living in damp or dirty places. It is mainly because of improvements in people's living conditions that childbirth has become so safe. Modern medicine has played a much smaller role.

This is not to say there are no benefits from having doctors and hospitals involved in childbirth. Ultrasound monitors, drugs to induce labor, forceps and suction to help babies to be born, and Cesarean sections all make childbirth safer for a small proportion of women. Without these procedures, childbirth would have been dangerous for them. For these women, technology can be life-saving.

Technology sometimes gets out of hand. Procedures that are useful for a small number of women can be applied to women who don't really need them. Induction rates in the 1970s climbed to as many as 60% of births in some hospitals. Women were being induced but not because their babies were at risk. Instead, they were induced because it was more convenient if they gave birth at certain times of the day or

115

Understanding Your Care in Labor

Before you agree to any medical procedure in labor, make sure you understand exactly why your doctor or midwife wants to do it and what it involves. Your mind will be much more at ease during your labor. You will feel better afterward if you have had all your questions answered.

The Questions to Ask

- What are the benefits for me and my baby?
- Are there any risks?
- What exactly does the procedure involve?
- If I agree to it, is it likely that I will need to have other interventions during my labor?

- Is there anything else we could try before doing this?
- What could happen if I decide to wait a little before making up my mind?
- What might happen if I decide not to go ahead with this procedure?

on certain days of the week. Cesarean-section rates climbed, too. A Cesarean section is only needed in about one in seven births. But in the United States, nearly one woman in four has a Cesarean section. And in some hospitals, it's closer to one woman in two! In Canada, almost 18% of all deliveries are Cesarean sections. This is clearly a crazy state of affairs. Each intervention in the natural process of giving birth carries a certain amount of risk. When interventions are used for women who don't need them, they can cause more harm than good.

Over the last few years, women's groups and healthcare providers have joined together to question some of the interventions that had become routine in childbirth. Books have been written that show, for instance, that for most women it is no safer to have a baby in the hospital than at home. Electronic monitors are no better at detecting babies in distress in labor than less intrusive methods, such as a Doppler or an ear trumpet. Breaking the bag of waters around the baby in order to speed up labor is only likely to reduce the length of labor by about half an hour. More and more research has shown how safe birth is and how harmful it can be to interfere with its natural process. As a result, people are beginning to swing away from interfering with labor.

Midwives tend to protect the woman in labor from unneeded interventions. They are likely to encourage her to trust her own body and to cope on her own. More and more women recognize that they are quite able to cope with labor. They understand that they do not need to behave like patients, lying on a hospital bed while they give birth. Instead, they can act like normal, healthy adults. They can choose to do what makes them feel best. They can remain upright and move about in labor. They can give birth to their babies kneeling, or squatting or on all fours.

Today we also know a lot more about how emotions govern the process of labor. If the mother is frightened and tense, her labor may slow and become more difficult. She is likely to have a much easier time if she has good support. She should be kept informed about how her labor is going and should be consulted about her care.

Magazines about birth and parenting urge women to decide for themselves about what happens in labor based on what they prefer and the knowledge they receive from healthcare providers. Women now have the chance to take an active role in the birth of their babies. This is both rewarding and frightening. But parenthood is all about making decisions for our children. It makes sense to start making those decisions when our babies are still in the uterus or while they are being born.

When women decide with their healthcare providers about their labor, what might have seemed an unwanted intervention at one time becomes something they have chosen:

"An intervention is something that's done to you without your consent. If I want to have a Cesarean section, that's not an intervention. Or if I want to have an epidural, that's not an intervention. To me, an intervention means things being taken out of your control or something that you're pressured into having."

"Even if you have interventions, you can still maintain some control if you've talked them over first."

Interventions in Labor

- *Induction of labor*—having your labor started by the doctor or nurse.
- *Vaginal exam (VE)*—when the doctor or nurse puts her fingers into the vagina to see how far open the cervix is. She can also learn what position the baby is in.
- *Artificial rupture of membranes (ARM)*—having the bag of waters broken.
- *Acceleration of labor*—using an intravenous drip to make contractions stronger. (Hormones to speed up labor may also be given by mouth.)
- *Fetal monitoring*—being monitored by machine. There are two types. Two transducers are strapped onto your abdomen, *or* an electrode is inserted into the baby's scalp.
- *Assisted delivery with forceps or ventouse*—using forceps or suction to help deliver the baby.
- *Cesarean section*—ECS–elective Cesarean section, or LSCS–lower-segment Cesarean section.

Women are wise enough to know that sometimes interventions are needed. They are not likely to make choices that put either themselves or their babies at risk: *"I don't see forceps and stitches—all those kinds of things—as problems if they're needed. I'll accept them if they're needed. I'll just regard them as part of the process of helping the baby out safely."*

"I want as natural a birth as possible. But if the baby's in distress and I understand why they want to do something, I'll go along with what they say. I'll be happy with that."

The mother is the person with the greatest interest in her baby's well-being. The choices she makes will reflect the concern that no harm should come to her child. Few women will choose to go against what healthcare providers recommend if they are given reasons for the advice they are being offered. And most women feel much better about their care if they have been consulted about it.

Induction—Getting Information

In some places, women used to be induced when they were exactly forty weeks pregnant or just a few days over their due date. Views about induction have changed. Most doctors now feel it's safe for a woman to go at least two weeks late (to 42 weeks). There are all sorts of ways of finding out if the baby is still doing well in the womb. And if he is, there seems little reason to disturb him. Most women will have given birth to their babies by 42 weeks of pregnancy, and nearly all of them by 43 weeks.

But doctors still have their own views about when a woman's labor should be induced: *"The nurse told me that one of the doctors here prefers to induce when you're a week late, more so than the others."*

The fact that opinions vary suggests that the choice about induction is often not clear-cut. So there is no reason why *your* opinion shouldn't count, too. You may have very strong feelings one way or the other about the merits of a prolonged pregnancy: *"I think if the baby's not ready to come out, there's a reason. They come when they want to come, when they're ready. We should leave well enough alone unless the baby's not doing well."*

But it can seem like an endless wait for some women: *"My doctor said that he is happy to let his patients go over [their due date] by three weeks. I feel like tearing my hair out!"*

Some women are surprised to find they have a choice about whether to be induced: *"My doctor will let you go 10 days late and then he'll induce you. I didn't know I had any other choice."*

Of course, there are times when the healthcare providers and the mother are likely to feel that there is no choice. Induction may be needed because both the mother and the baby will be better off if the baby is born. A woman with very high blood pressure is one such example: *"Throughout my pregnancy, I had high blood pressure. I knew there was a danger to both me and the baby. So I was happy to be induced."*

Learning about induction sometimes depends on having the courage to ask questions: *"After we started asking questions, they offered us other options. But they didn't mention those until we started asking questions. In the end, I wasn't induced. I went thirteen days over."*

Not being given a reason for induction doesn't seem right to most women. Some will demand to be told: *"When induction was first mentioned, he just said 'Come in tomorrow,' and walked out of the room. I said, 'Excuse me!' It was a student doctor. As soon as I started to ask questions, he said, 'I'll have to get the obstetrician.' The OB came and was a little defensive to start with. We were saying things like, 'What happens if we aren't induced? Is there any other option? What other choices do we have?' In other words, we were trying to find out what we needed to know to make a decision. After a while I just said to him, 'Please just tell us all you can. Then can we have a few minutes to think about things on our own?' Once I calmed down, he did too. And he did tell us what we needed to know. We talked about it and he came back five minutes later and we told him our decision. He was OK with what we wanted and there was no shouting at all!"*

Very often, a calm but assertive approach works best to help you learn what you need to know. It can also help you build trust and respect with your healthcare providers.

Reasons Why Labor Might Be Induced

1. *The mother has gone over her due date by more than two weeks.* Induction used to be offered when the mother was just a few days past her due date. But most of the time it is now believed to be quite safe to wait until 42 weeks.

2. *Pre-eclampsia.* The mother's blood pressure is very high and she has protein in her urine.

3. *The baby seems to have stopped growing* and the mother is feeling fewer movements than she did before.

4. *The mother's waters have broken but contractions have not started.* Induction may be suggested because the mother's uterus or the baby could become infected from bacteria in the vagina. (Vaginal exams, after the waters have broken, can contribute to infections. They help bring bacteria from the vagina into the uterus. After the waters have broken, vaginal exams should be kept to a minimum.)

5. There are a number of other, less common, reasons for an induction:

   • The mother has given birth to a very large baby before and the doctors want to prevent this baby from growing as large.

   • The mother has had a very fast labor before. She wants to be sure that this labor takes place in a safe environment.

   • The mother has genital herpes or warts. The baby needs to be born at a time when the warts are not "active" or weepy.

   • The mother's baby has died inside the uterus. She doesn't want to wait for labor to start by itself.

Other ways to induce labor

There are ways to induce labor that you can try for yourself if you are well past your due date and don't want to be induced in a hospital. These are, in the words of one woman: *"Spicy food, hot bath, hot sex!"*

No research supports the first two ideas. But the last suggestion is well-founded. The semen the man ejaculates during love-making contains prostaglandins. Vaginal inserts of prostaglandins are often used to induce labor. Plus, breast stimulation causes a hormone to be released (oxytocin) that makes the uterus contract. Breast stimulation can bring on strong contractions in the last few weeks of pregnancy. This can help start labor.

What does it feel like to be induced?

You might be asked to come into the hospital the night before you are induced. Or you might already be in the hospital because you haven't been well. The night before labor is induced can be a very long one: *"When Steve went home, I felt very, very small there in the dark with everyone else asleep. I was awake all night and I wanted to go home."*

Induced labors are often hard and fast. Women find that instead of having time to adjust to a labor that builds slowly, they are plunged into very strong and frequent contractions right from the start: *"I was induced. The effect of the suppositories was nothing one minute— no labor at all. And then all of a sudden I had contractions lasting one minute or a minute and a half with thirty seconds off in between! I had been checked shortly before they started me and I wasn't dilated at all. In about three hours I went to 8cm. I had no idea what was going on. For me, it was a lot more traumatic than I thought it would be."*

Sometimes a woman is induced and nothing happens: *"I had the suppositories and George went home. I wasn't worried. I was just bored. Nothing happened."*

Sometimes the suppositories don't work until the second or third try. Or other methods may be needed to get contractions started.

How Is Labor Induced?

There are three methods:

- *Prostaglandin suppositories:* Suppositories are oval tablets of jelly that the doctor or nurse puts into the woman's vagina close to the cervix. Suppositories can help make the cervix "ripe." That is, they help make the cervix become soft and ready for labor. After the nurse has given the suppositories, the mother is monitored in bed for an hour or so. A belt is strapped to her abdomen to see if contractions are starting and how her baby reacts to them. (Prostaglandin can also be given in the form of a gel.)

- *Breaking the waters:* If the mother's cervix has opened a little, the doctor or midwife can use an amnihook. This looks like a very long crotchet hook. It's used to break the bag of waters around the baby. The mother lies on her back at the end of the bed with her knees drawn up and apart. She is often covered in green, sterile towels. The waters drain into a bucket placed beneath the bed.

- *A hormone drip:* The mother is given an IV drip that contains syntocinon, a synthetic hormone that makes the uterus contract. The amount of syntocinon given to the mother is slowly increased to mimic the buildup of oxytocin in a normal labor.

Induced labors can be a lot more painful than labors that start on their own. Even with good support, women sometimes need more help from drugs to cope with the pain of an induced labor:

"If I were induced again, I would definitely have another epidural. I couldn't cope without one."

"The suppositories didn't work, so they set up an IV drip. I felt I just went bang—right into heavy labor. I wanted an epidural the next minute."

Induced labors end in emergency Cesareans more often than normal labors do. Sometimes an induced labor leads to other interventions. This has been called *the cascade of intervention: "I had the suppositories. Then they broke my waters because they said it might speed up labor, which it didn't. It didn't do anything. Then I was all hooked up to the monitors. I was in so much pain, I had to have the epidural. By this time, the baby was showing some signs of distress. So then they thought that since I wasn't dilating, I needed a Cesarean."*

Some women are happy to be induced. They are pleased that the long days of waiting after their due date has passed are coming to an end: *"They gave me the prostaglandin gel Sunday night. I was told that nothing would happen overnight and it didn't, except for a mild backache. Then they gave me more at eight in the morning and monitored me for half an hour. At ten the contractions started getting stronger and stronger. I went into full labor, which I thought was going to last for hours and hours. But she was born at twenty to eleven, so it was great. I would be induced again if I was late. There are pros and cons. I was very lucky that it all went quickly, and I only had to have gel."*

Other Methods of Intervention

Speeding up labor

In some hospitals, it is common for women to have their waters broken during labor. The reason often given for this is that it will speed up labor. Or an IV drip with synthetic oxytocin may be started to make the woman's contractions stronger and to open her cervix faster. When you talk to women who have given birth, it can be surprising to learn just how many have had these kinds of procedures. You may feel that it isn't likely that nature requires so much help. It can be very tough

Pre-eclampsia (Pregnancy-induced Hypertension—PIH)

What is it?
A disease of pregnancy.

What are the signs and symptoms?
• Protein in the urine

• High blood pressure

• Headaches and spots before the eyes

• Sickness (nausea)

• Pain in the top half of the abdomen

Each of the last three symptoms could also be caused by some other reason. But contact your doctor or midwife at once if you experience any of them. The symptoms might mean you have very serious pre-eclampsia and require urgent medical care.

How do I know if I've got it?
Each time you have a prenatal check-up, your urine will be checked to see if there is protein in it. The nurse will also take your blood pressure. These tests help your healthcare providers find out if you have pre-eclampsia or are at risk for it.

What are the problems for me and my baby if I have pre-eclampsia?
If your blood pressure is high, the placenta doesn't work well. Your baby may not get all the food and oxygen he needs to grow properly. Sometimes with high blood pressure, the placenta can detach from the uterus (this is rare). If that happens, the baby would almost certainly be lost. The mother would be at risk, too, from loss of blood. Very high blood pressure is also bad for you because it can damage your kidneys. It can also cause you to have seizures (but this is rare, too).

What will happen if I get pre-eclampsia?
Your doctor or midwife may want to see you more often to check your blood pressure and test your urine. She is likely to refer you for nutrition assessment and education. If she doesn't, ask her about it. Or find a dietitian on your own with whom you can work. Nutrition education has been shown to improve the birthweight of infants whose mothers had pre-eclampsia.

You may be told to rest at home. Or you may be asked to come to the hospital to rest, though there's no proof that resting helps pre-eclampsia. If your pre-eclampsia is very bad, you may have your labor induced. Or, you may be given a Cesarean section. This makes sure your baby can be born before either of you comes to any harm.

for a woman in labor to challenge the system. You may not be sure whether, in your case, the procedure might really be needed for you and your baby:

"Of ten women I knew, all had babies at the same time. Nine of them ended up having a drip to speed up labor. Now, I don't believe that was really needed. But one out of ten might be needed. And how do you know you are not that one?"

Active Labor Management

What is it?

In Ireland in the 1960s, a now-famous obstetrician named Kieran O'Driscoll noticed that the longer a labor lasted, the more likely it was that problems would arise. So he tried to find a way to manage labor that would ensure that all the women coming to his hospital gave birth in twelve hours or less.

He used a graph to chart how quickly the mother's cervix opened. If it was opening slowly, her labor was speeded up. He would either break the waters around the baby or give her a hormone drip to strengthen contractions. Because the progress of labor needed to be observed with care, a nurse or a midwife was assigned to each woman to be with her throughout her labor until her baby was born.

Many hospitals throughout the world have followed O'Driscoll's plan. Check to see if your hospital follows the practice of Active Labor Management. Active Management has benefits, but also many drawbacks.

Benefits:

- Some women are relieved to know that they will not be allowed to labor longer than a certain length of time. They are happy to accept a Cesarean section or forceps birth if labor lasts longer than agreed.
- The support offered by a nurse who stays with the mother throughout her labor is tremendous. The nurse often helps the mother cope well with a labor that has been made stronger or faster.

Drawbacks:

- Shorter labors may not be easier to cope with than longer ones. If the mother can relax and has good support, she will often cope well with a labor that is slow. When contractions build slowly, she has time to get used to their increasing strength.
- Not all women (or healthcare providers) are happy with the thought of interfering with a normal labor simply to make it faster.
- Speeding up the labor through the use of hormones may mean that the mother needs to use more drugs for pain than she would have otherwise.
- Because active labor management often involves the mother having a drip in her arm and being monitored at all times, she may not be able to move around. This may make labor more painful and difficult.
- Hospitals looking to cut costs may practice active labor management, but assign one nurse or midwife to care for a number of women at the same time. In such cases, the nurse depends a great deal on the monitor output. The mother is left to labor alone for most of the time.

It's always good to ask if you're not certain why a procedure is being suggested. Your peace of mind both during labor and afterward will be much greater if you understand the reasons why things were done. Healthcare providers are busy people. Sometimes they don't remember that something they think of as routine might make no sense to you.

You will nearly always find that if you ask questions, you will get answers: *"I asked things like, 'What's in the drip?' I was worried about side effects. They were very good and they did tell me. But they didn't offer to tell me. You always have to ask."*

Talk things over with your doctor. If you both agree it could help to have your waters broken, you are much more likely to be happy with the outcome: *"They broke my waters. That was the best thing the doctor could have done. My cervix had been stuck at 3cm. Afterwards, it jumped to 7cm. The doctor did it for a reason, which we'd discussed and I'd agreed to."*

As with other interventions, having your waters broken could in itself cause problems: *"I think they tried to break the waters too soon and that's why it didn't work. Later they did it successfully. I am sure that it was because of having my waters broken that I got a uterine infection. The doctor who did it had a bad cold. It meant I went home on antibiotics. And I had to go back three weeks later to have more antibiotics with an IV drip."*

Speeding Up Labor

Your doctor may suggest breaking the waters around the baby to speed up labor. This is called *acceleration of labor*. The doctor may also want to break the waters to see what color they are. If they are dark or green, this could mean that your baby is not coping well with labor.

Here are some points you might want to think about:

• The bag of waters is designed to act as a buffer zone around your baby. It protects him from the strength of the contractions. Once this buffer zone has been taken away, your baby may find labor much more stressful.

• Research has found that breaking the waters only shortens labor by about half an hour.

• Some women find contractions are much harder for a while after the waters are broken. Kneeling with your shoulders lower than your bottom can help for the first contraction or two.

Monitors

We live in an age of technology. We use technology at home and at work. Many women find comfort in the thought of their baby's heart being monitored by machine during labor. The baby's heartbeat is fast—twice the rate of your own—and not always regular. It is quite an addictive sound: *"I had the belt monitor on and they said, 'Do you want to take it off?' I think they always put it on when you first go into labor for fifteen minutes or so, just to check and learn what the norm is. By*

Monitors in Labor

What does it mean to monitor labor?

Sometimes it is easy to forget that labor is something the baby has to go through as well as the mother. Just as the mother may sometimes find labor hard to cope with, so may her baby.

The nurse listens to your baby's heartbeat with a stethoscope or Doppler. Or she looks at the pattern of his heartbeat on a monitor printout. These help her understand how your baby is being affected by contractions. When your uterus contracts, your baby's umbilical cord is squeezed and his oxygen supply is reduced. His heartbeat changes when there is less oxygen.

Most babies cope well with contractions, and their heartbeat returns quickly to normal after each one. A few find labor very stressful. Their heartbeats become weaker.

If it seems to the doctor or midwife that your baby's heartbeat is too slow during contractions, or takes too long to return to a normal rate between them, they may believe a Cesarean section is the safest way for your baby to be born.

Statement by the American College of Obstetrics and Gynecology

In 1989, the American College of Obstetrics and Gynecology (ACOG) stated, "It is now increasingly evident from available data that EFM (electronic fetal monitoring) has no inherent benefit over intermittent auscultation in both high- and low-risk patients." *Intermittent auscultation* means checking the baby's heart tones from time to time throughout labor with a stethoscope or a Doppler.

---

that stage, I had gotten used to hearing the baby's heart. I loved hearing it. That was the only intervention I had, just the belt. I had thought I wouldn't want anything. But I did like having the belt on . . . listening to my baby racehorse!"

When a baby has a problem or is being born too soon, the mother may be reassured to see from the printout on the monitor that she is all right: *"I had a lot of intervention. But I knew that it was because the baby came so early. I was glad to have it all, even the monitor. Just watching that heartbeat, knowing she was healthy, was helpful. I needed to know. It really helped."*

But some women find that watching the monitor makes them more anxious that something may go wrong:

"I found it better not to watch the monitor. I just thought, 'Well, what's got to happen will happen.' I asked for it to be turned down, and I didn't look at it."

Electronic Monitors

What's good about them:

• The doctor or nurse can see clearly how your baby's heartbeat responds to contractions.

• A nurse can consult a doctor if your baby appears to find labor stressful.

• Electronic monitors reassure many mothers, fathers and healthcare providers.

What's *not* so good about them:

• Printouts from monitors are not always accurate. This depends on the quality of the machine being used and on how often it has been serviced.

• It is not easy to interpret readings of a baby's heartbeat in labor. Even highly qualified doctors and nurses may not agree about what a certain reading means. Someone with less training may not notice or understand important readings.

• Because monitor readings are hard to understand, some women will have emergency Cesarean sections when their babies are perfectly all right.

• Having a monitor on her abdomen or an electrode in the baby's scalp often means that the mother has to stay in bed. A woman copes best with labor when she can be upright and is free to move around. Both she and her baby are much more likely to become distressed if she cannot move freely. So monitors may cause the distress the machine records!

• Some parents worry that a fetal scalp electrode hurts their baby when it is inserted into the baby's scalp.

• Research (and there has been a lot of it) does not suggest that monitors make labor safer for babies. Babies who are not monitored do just as well. If a monitor suggests that a baby is distressed, this should be confirmed in other ways. The oxygen levels in a sample of blood taken from the baby's scalp should be checked before deciding to do a Cesarean section.

"They monitored the baby all the way through. I got really scared at the end. I didn't understand what the monitor meant and I thought the baby might die."

With monitors, the mother is often confined to a bed or to a chair. Not being able to move around may lead to a long, painful labor. In the end, the baby may need help to be born. This is an instance of the cascade of intervention: *"I couldn't move around because of the monitors. I got very, very tired and it was so painful. I don't know how long I was in second stage. I remember pushing for a long time. The forceps and the episiotomy were not what I had wanted at all."*

Different Kinds of Monitors

There are different kinds of monitors. You might want to think about which sort you would prefer. If you are having your baby at home, the midwife will monitor your baby's heartbeat using one of these methods:

- *An ear trumpet* (Pinard's stethoscope). This is a cone-shaped piece of plastic or metal that the midwife places on your abdomen. It helps her listen to your baby's heartbeat with her ear.

- *A hand-held Doppler* (Sonicaid®). This is a kind of small ultrasound machine. The midwife places what looks like a microphone on your abdomen. Both of you can hear the baby's heartbeat.

If you are having your baby in a birth center or hospital, you can have your baby's heartbeat monitored with either of the methods described above. Or you can use one of these methods:

- *Belt monitor.* Two round ultrasound monitors are placed on your abdomen. One is placed at the top of your belly, which is where contractions start. The other is placed over your baby's heart.

The transducers are held in place by an elastic belt. A wire from each transducer goes to a machine placed next to your chair or bed. You must be very still. The machine gives a printout of your baby's heartbeat and of your contractions. The midwife uses the readings to assess how well your baby is coping with labor.

- *Fetal-scalp electrode.* This is a monitor the doctor inserts into your baby's scalp after your waters have broken. The electrode is shaped like a small coil, which is sharp at one end. This more or less screws a little way into the baby's scalp. A wire from the monitor passes down your vagina and is attached to a machine. The machine prints out a record of your baby's heartbeat. The fetal-scalp electrode may be used with an abdominal transducer that also records your contractions.

- *Fetal-blood sampling.* The doctor or midwife can take blood from your baby's scalp during labor to check his oxygen levels. This gives your caregivers more data about how your baby is coping with labor.

Belt monitor

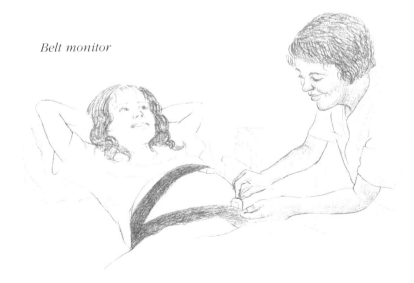

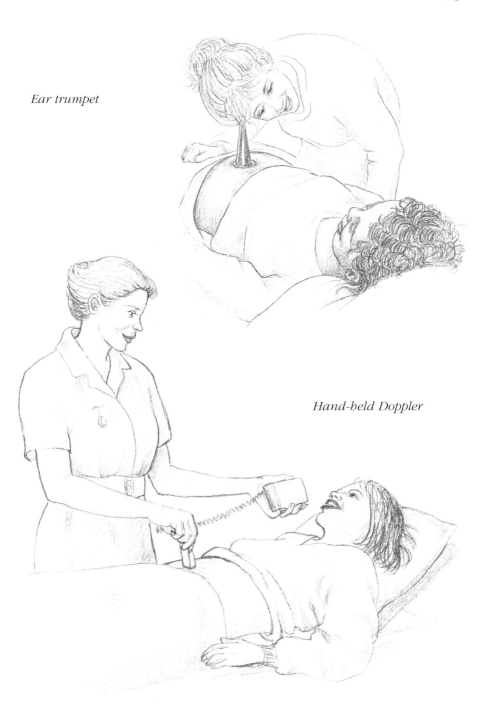

Ear trumpet

Hand-held Doppler

Perineal Massage

Little research has been done into whether massage of the perineum (the place between the vagina and the back passage, or rectum) in pregnancy helps the woman prevent a tear when she has her baby. A lot of women are convinced that it is helpful. Perineal massage is a simple technique that you carry out once a day for the last few weeks of pregnancy.

- Use a lubricating jelly. Try KY jelly, which you can get from a drug store. Or you could use a scent-free oil, such as almond or olive oil. Put one finger just inside the vagina. Gently move it across the rim of the vagina at the back.

- After a few days, try inserting two fingers.

- Soon, you or your partner may be able to insert five fingers. Open them gently until you feel a stretching sensation. When you feel this, hold the stretch for a few seconds and then let go. Work up to a few minutes of stretching and then releasing daily.

- Remember that the perineum is designed by nature to stretch.

Episiotomy

Many pregnant women worry about being cut at the back wall of the vagina during labor. This is done to enlarge the opening and help out the baby. Episiotomy is one of the most common surgical procedures performed. But in fact, often it is not needed. There is no doubt that cutting this most private part of a woman's body can change the way she feels about herself: *"I wish someone had told me beforehand what it feels like to have had an episiotomy. I don't feel the same any more. I feel different. Do all mothers feel different down below afterward?"*

"My episiotomy healed. But I can't say I'll ever be back to normal, or I'll ever feel normal. It didn't feel good to wear jeans for a long time. Not that it hurts. It's not painful, it's just that I don't feel quite right. I don't know if it's all in my mind, but it just doesn't feel right."

For some women, having an episiotomy is not traumatic. How you feel may depend on the way you were cut, the way you were sewn, and how you were treated: *"They had the birth plan, which said I would rather not have an episiotomy. But they asked if they could do a very small cut. I didn't have strong feelings about it at that point and it was fine."*

If you have an episiotomy or tear during labor, you are likely to need stitches after the birth. Some women will heal quickly without any problem. But for others, healing can be a long, slow process. There has been little research into how women can reduce their risk of tearing. But many women believe that massage of the perineum (the place

Episiotomies and Tears

Help yourself prevent tears or the need for an episiotomy

An episiotomy is a cut in the back wall of the vagina at the outlet. It makes the opening wider and helps the baby be born more quickly. Women are anxious that a cut or tear in the vagina or the skin between the vagina and the rectum (the perineum) will make having sex painful. They worry that it may leave scars, look bad or make it hard to use a tampon. Women who have been sexually abused may find the thought of a cut frightening. It can bring back memories of damage they have suffered to their sexual parts when they were abused.

There are things you can do to reduce your risk of tearing or needing a cut during labor.

- Try pushing in an upright position. Don't sit on your tailbone. Your pelvis will open wider. In this position you will give your baby as much room as possible. The easier it is for your baby to be born, the less strain he will put on your vagina and perineum.

- Relax your vagina to allow your baby to come through. Don't hold back.

- When the doctor tells you that the baby's head will be born with the next contraction, get down on all fours. Then your baby's head will come out slowly from the vagina. This permits the perineum to stretch gently over his face. Such a gentle birth protects the delicate blood vessels inside your baby's head from damage. It also protects you from tearing, by giving your tissues time to stretch.

- The doctor may tell you to pant rather than push when your baby's head is being born. This will also help to slow the birth and make it more gentle.

between the vagina and the back passage) in pregnancy and pelvic-floor-muscle exercise will help them give birth safely:

"I'm doing perineal massage like crazy. I hope it's going to help."

"I didn't do the massage last time but I did a lot of pelvic-floor-muscle exercise. Learning to relax the muscles is very useful when the baby's being born. I didn't have a cut or any bruising."

Be sure to tell your doctor or midwife if you don't want to have an episiotomy. Then he can work with you to achieve a gentle birth: *"I said to her that my biggest fear was an episiotomy. I was terrified about that. I told her, and she really did go out of her way to ensure that I didn't need one. She tried all kinds of things. She put a hot washcloth on the perineum just when Lucy was being born. And she had me give birth on all fours so that the baby's head would come out slowly. There are ways to prevent tears. I found the midwives were very helpful."*

Forceps and ventouse (suction)

Sometimes the birth of a baby can be difficult: *"The midwife kept telling the doctor to go away. She said I'd be able to push this baby out without forceps. But another half hour went by and I was still pushing. The doctor came back in again and I felt it wasn't working. In fact, the baby was stuck. The head hadn't turned."*

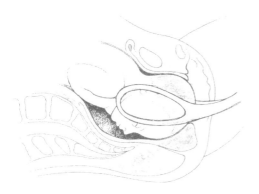

A forceps birth

At times like this it may be safer for the mother and the baby if they are given some help. Often a forceps birth means just lifting the baby out of the vagina: *"Ben's head had already dropped down low. So it was just a question of pulling him out the last little bit. I tried to push and take part in the birth."*

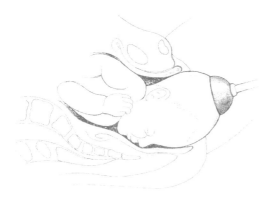

A ventouse birth

Unless the baby needs to be born quickly, ventouse (suction) births can be kinder for mothers than forceps. They do less damage to the vagina. You can often choose whether you would prefer to have forceps or suction: *"I asked to have suction instead of forceps. I was lucky that the doctor who was on call was a specialist in ventouse. I didn't want any part of the metal forceps."*

Ventouse can also be used even before the mother has started pushing in the second stage of labor: *"I had suction because I had the belt monitor in the first stage. It showed that each time I had a contraction, the baby's heart rate slowed down. I said, 'Is this going to be a Cesarean section?' But when they checked me, the baby's*

Forceps and Ventouse

A baby sometimes needs extra help to be born. The mother may be exhausted after a long labor. Her contractions and pushing may become weaker as the second stage of labor continues. The baby himself may have become stressed by his efforts to be born. Or he may not be in the best position to be born. He could need help to turn into a better position so that he can come into the world more easily. In all these cases, the mother may be offered forceps or ventouse to help.

Forceps come in pairs. Each part has a curved blade and a handle. They are applied carefully. One goes on either side of the baby's head and the handles fit together. The doctor asks the mother to push when she has her next contraction. Then he pulls at the same time. Sometimes, the doctor needs to pull very firmly. This can look frightening to labor-support persons.

The ventouse looks a little like a plunger with a plastic cup at the end. This is placed on the top of the baby's head. Suction is applied either by hand or with a pump. The baby's scalp is sucked into the cap. It takes six or seven minutes for the suction to work. The doctor can then pull the baby out of the vagina helped by the mother's own pushing efforts. Sometimes the cap comes off the baby's head and needs to be put on again.

Which should you choose?

These are some points to think about:

- Is your doctor skilled at using forceps? How about ventouse? It's good to find out during your prenatal checkups whether both forceps and ventouse births are possible.

- A forceps birth often can be carried out quickly. If your baby needs to be born in a couple of minutes, this is the better option. A ventouse birth will take up to 10 minutes. Time is needed for the suction to work on the baby's head.

- Ventouse births are far kinder for *mothers*. The suction cap takes up much less room in the vagina and causes far less damage than a pair of metal forceps. You often don't need an episiotomy with a ventouse birth. You *always* need an episiotomy for a forceps birth. Research suggests that for the baby, there may not be much difference between forceps and ventouse. But the mother will almost always have much less pain and trouble after a ventouse birth.

head was right there. And I was fully dilated. They used the ventouse. On the second try, she came out fast."

And sometimes the ventouse cap won't stay on the baby's head. Then forceps are the only choice: *"The doctor tried ventouse with me first and it kept slipping off. So he said, 'I'm sorry, I have to use the forceps.' But, as it happened, Sam didn't have a mark on him afterwards."*

Stitches and Healing

When the birth is managed slowly, many women who are not having their first babies won't tear or need to be cut. But many first-time mothers do suffer at least small tears. And quite a few have an episiotomy. There are all sorts of things you can do to feel better while you are healing.

- Practice your pelvic-floor-muscle exercises without fail a few times each day. These can speed up the healing process.

- Eat plenty of fiber-rich foods, such as:
  - whole-grain bread
  - cereal with bran
  - potatoes with their skins
  - fruit with the skin on
  - green leafy vegetables

  These prevent constipation so you won't strain your stitches.

- Keep a pillow with you so you always have something soft to sit on.

- It is *not* true that salt baths will help heal your stitches. But they can be very soothing. If you find that salt dries your skin, try using a saltwater douche. Boil some water and then allow it to cool. It should feel warm against your skin, but not hot. Stir in a tablespoonful of salt. Then sit on the toilet. Pour the salt solution between your legs from front to back so that it bathes your stitches.

- If you are going to have a bath in the hospital, make sure it is clean. If it doesn't look very clean, tell the nurse, but don't use it. Most after-childbirth infections are caught in hospitals!

- The homeopathic remedy, arnica, helps heal a bruised perineum and soothes the pain of stitches.

If your stitches are still sore many days after the birth, be sure to let your doctor or midwife know. Don't suffer in silence. Your body is too important. When you start making love again, if you find that intercourse is painful, see your doctor. It should not hurt to make love after giving birth!

Emergency Cesarean

When you expect to have a normal birth, it can be frightening to find that things are going wrong and that your baby needs to be born quickly by Cesarean. There can be a feeling of panic in the room. Lots of people may come and go. And there's the mother in the middle of it all, fearful for the safety of her child:

"They put me on a drip to speed up the contractions. Then his heartbeat started going down. It took longer and longer in between each contraction to recover. It was awful! That's when you want them to do something. I was in a real panic. The doctor was, too. She went to get the anesthetist. And I was saying, 'Get this baby out of me. Just give me a Cesarean. I want him out.'"

For other women, the decision to do a Cesarean is far more calm. Then they can better understand what is going on: *"They did consult with us all the way. They told us what was happening. I felt fully involved, which was very positive. It wasn't like they just decided to do the C-section and that was it."*

"I had an emergency Cesarean. But the nurse explained to me what was happening. That helped me calm down a little, and that was very good."

"I had an epidural Cesarean. The anesthetist took great care to tell me exactly what he was doing and why and how I would feel."

Elective Cesarean

An elective Cesarean is one that has been planned to take place before the woman goes into labor: *"The doctor was very gentle and kind. He said, 'Well, I think you're going to see this baby a little sooner than you'd expected.' We talked about how quickly I needed to have the Cesarean. He came up to the maternity ward to see me and the baby afterward. I thought he was really good."*

Many women choose to have an epidural anesthetic for their Cesarean. Then they can be awake to greet their baby when he is born. Their labor-support person can also be with them. It is not always possible to choose between an epidural and a general anesthetic if you need an emergency Cesarean. But in most cases, you can choose to have an epidural if your Cesarean is planned: *"I had an epidural for the Cesarean. Phil was with me. After the baby was born, we held her together while they sewed me up."*

If the woman is not able to hold her baby herself as soon as he is born, she can see her partner or labor-support person holding him: *"He was with me when I had the C-section. He ended up holding the baby first, which was really good."*

Finding out why you needed a Cesarean

A Cesarean section is a major abdominal surgery. Most women will need a few weeks and often months to recover from it. There is little doubt that a woman recovers more quickly if her mind is at ease because she knows why her Cesarean was needed. She should know,

Cesarean Birth

There are two kinds of Cesarean section:

- *Elective*—This means the mother and her doctor have planned and prepared for a Cesarean before labor starts.

- *Emergency*—This means that a sudden decision is made to perform a Cesarean because a problem has come up.

Reasons for an elective Cesarean

- The baby is thought to be too big to go through the mother's pelvis.

- The placenta is lying across the cervix and prevents the baby from getting out.

- The baby is lying across the uterus rather than head or bottom down. In this position, a vaginal birth isn't possible.

- The mother is carrying twins, triplets or more babies (but twins don't always have to be born by Cesarean section).

- The baby is thought to be too weak to go through labor.

- The mother has severe pre-eclampsia. Her baby needs to be born quickly both for his and her sakes.

- The baby is lying in the womb in the breech position. (His bottom is coming first rather than his head.)

- The mother has an active case of genital herpes or warts. She must have a Cesarean section to prevent the baby from getting infected.

You don't always have to have a Cesarean if your baby is in the breech position. It may be possible to have a normal vaginal birth. But many doctors do not suggest that first-time mothers have a vaginal birth for a breech baby.

You need to discuss with your doctor whether she thinks you should have a Cesarean or a vaginal birth and why.

Reasons for an emergency Cesarean

- The mother has an illness, such as diabetes, that complicates her labor.

- The baby's heartbeat shows that he is not coping well with labor. The doctor describes this as the baby being "distressed." Another sign of distress (sometimes) is green or dark waters around the baby. This means the baby has moved his bowels in the womb. This is called having *meconium-stained waters*.

- The umbilical cord comes through the cervix before the baby. When the cord is trapped between the baby's head (or bottom) and the cervix, the baby's life-line is cut off.

- The doctor has tried to help the baby to be born by using forceps or the ventouse, but neither has worked. The only choice left is Cesarean.

- The cervix opens a little but then doesn't any more, even after many hours of labor.

- After the cervix is fully open, the baby does not move down through the pelvis despite the mother's pushing. This may be because the baby does not have his head tucked in closely to his body.

These last two are often called *failure to progress* even though there is no failure on either the baby's or the mother's part. Sometimes there seems to be no reason why the cervix doesn't open fully, or why the baby isn't born in the second stage of labor. When you have a problem like this in your first labor it doesn't mean that it will happen again next time.

Your Choices for a Cesarean

- Do you want to have a spinal anesthetic, an epidural or a general anesthetic?
- Do you want your labor-support person to stay with you the whole time? (This may not be possible if you are having a general anesthetic. Ask the doctor or nurse.)

If you are awake for the Cesarean:

- Do you want the doctor to tell you what is happening?
- Do you want to see the operation? If so, ask to have the screen removed.
- Do you want to find out the sex of your baby for yourself rather than having the doctor tell you?
- Do you want to hold your baby right away, while you are still on the operating table?

- If your baby is well, do you want him to stay with you until the operation is over? Do you want to keep him with you when you go to the recovery room?
- Do you want to breast-feed your baby while you are still on the operating table?

If you are asleep for the operation:

- Do you want your baby to be given to your partner to hold as soon as possible?
- Do you want someone to take a photo of your baby being born?
- Do you want your baby to be bottle-fed by the nurses during the first hours after your operation?

too, if she decides to have another baby, whether she is likely to need a Cesarean next time also. Not knowing the reason for the Cesarean can cause ongoing distress: *"A lot of my feelings about the Cesarean came long afterward. Now it's still a problem for me. What on earth was going on?"*

It is crucial that the mother not go home with her new baby without a thorough explanation: *"I asked to go through my chart so that I knew exactly why I'd needed the section. The midwife was very helpful. She went through the chart with a fine-tooth comb. That was really important."*

Sometimes it seems that you can't learn what you need to know: *"I asked a resident doctor about seeing my chart. I wanted to know why they'd done the Cesarean. I didn't know what had happened. And he said, 'Oh that's not possible. You'll have to write to the hospital.' I said, 'I'm not attacking what you've done. I just want to know.' But they wouldn't tell me."*

To Be Awake or Not to Be Awake?

If your baby needs to be born quickly by emergency Cesarean, you may be offered a general anesthetic. This can be given more quickly than anything else. If you are having an elective Cesarean, or you need a Cesarean during labor but there's no rush, you can often choose whether you want to be awake or asleep when your baby is born. Being awake means having either an epidural or a spinal anesthetic.

Epidural/Spinal

What's good about it

- You will be awake to see and hold your baby as soon as he is born. You will probably be able to cuddle him while the operation is being finished.

- Your labor-support person will be able to stay with you in the operating room. The two of you will share the first moments of your baby's life.

- Women lose less blood when they have an epidural rather than a general anesthetic for a Cesarean. So you should recover more quickly afterwards.

What's not so good about it

- Some women are terrified at the thought of being awake while they are having major surgery. If you are one of these, you will feel better with a general anesthetic.

- The noises and smells of the operating room can be frightening. So can the pulling and tugging that you feel while your baby is being delivered.

General Anesthetic

What's good about it

- You will sleep through the whole operation and know nothing about it.

What's not so good about it

- You will sleep through the whole operation and know nothing about it.

- You will not be awake to greet your baby when he is born. You may feel groggy for quite a few hours after the operation is over. It could be a while before you hold your baby for the first time.

- Your partner or labor-support person will almost certainly not be able to be with you.

- Blood loss is greater after a general-anesthetic Cesarean. You may recover more slowly than after an epidural Cesarean. There also seems to be a higher risk of feeling depressed after the birth.

- Research suggests that babies born with a general anesthetic develop more slowly.

If this happens, try asking a more senior doctor or the nurse who was with you during labor to discuss the Cesarean with you. You have a legal right to see your chart. If you have any trouble getting your questions answered, ask to speak to the Chief of Obstetric Services.

You need to be able to understand what happened during labor and the events leading up to the operation. It will help you feel good about the way in which your baby was born and about yourself:

"I wasn't upset because I knew exactly why it had happened."

What Happens When You Have a Cesarean

Most hospitals can prepare a mother for a Cesarean. They can deliver her baby within ten minutes of deciding that she needs to have an emergency birth! It takes a lot longer to stitch you up again. You can expect the operation to continue for about 40 minutes after the birth of your baby.

• Either you, or your labor-support person if you are not well enough, signs a consent form for the operation.

• If this is an elective Cesarean, you may be given two rectal inserts a few hours before the operation. These help you empty your bowels. You will be asked not to eat anything after a certain time.

• The top half of your pubic hair is shaved.

• You put on a hospital gown. Any jewelry that you do not wish to take off, such as a wedding ring, is covered with tape. You are asked to wash off your makeup, remove nail polish and take out your contact lenses or dentures if you wear them.

• You may be given a small amount of medicine to drink. This will neutralize the acid in your stomach. Then if any acid should pass into your lungs during the operation, it will not cause damage.

• Your bladder may be emptied with a catheter. Often this is done after the anesthetic has been given. Then you won't feel the midwife putting the thin plastic tube into your bladder.

• An IV drip is put into your arm.

• You are given a general anesthetic, a spinal, or an epidural anesthetic. If you already have an epidural in place, this is topped up so that it is working fully.

• Women who are awake during their Cesarean describe feeling strange pulling and pushing sensations in their abdomen. These are not painful. But they can be scary if you don't expect them.

"People's first reaction when they hear you've had a C-section is, 'Oh no. What a shame.' But I'm saying, 'No, no. It's not a shame! I know it had to be that way. He's here and he's fine and it's OK.'"

Asking Questions

It is important to understand what is happening in labor. It helps if you can communicate well with the medical and nursing staff. Not knowing what is going on causes additional stress for the woman. This can increase the chance of things going wrong during the birth:

What to Expect the First Few Days after a Cesarean

- You may have a lot of pain. Ask for an injection or tablets to control the pain for as long as you need them. You now have a tiny baby to get to know and care for and enjoy. You can't do any of these things if you are in pain.

- You will not be allowed to have anything to eat or drink for quite a while after your operation. The IV drip in your arm ensures that you do not become dehydrated. Many women feel very hungry after the birth of their baby. They find it hard to wait until they can have a snack.

- A physical therapist may visit you soon after your operation. She will show you how to cough to keep your chest clear. She will also help you get out of bed and walk around. Despite your worst fears, you will not split in half! The sooner you walk around, the less likely you are to have the severe gas pains that often follow abdominal surgery.

- For a day or two after the operation, you may have a catheter in your bladder. You may also have a drain coming from your incision, which empties into a bottle. It's hard to take a catheter bag and drainage bottle with you wherever you go. But it's still important to get up and move around.

- A nurse will show you how to hold your baby or lie with him beside you so that you can nurse without hurting your abdomen. Yes, you can breast-feed your baby after a Cesarean. You can be given painkillers that will not harm him if they are absorbed into your milk.

- How will you *feel* after your Cesarean? Some women just feel very, very happy that their baby has been born safely. Some may go through an anxious and lonely time because their baby is in intensive care. And some, who have their baby with them, feel unhappy that they were not able to have a vaginal birth. All these feelings are normal and to be respected. You might find it helpful to talk to your doctor about the Cesarean and why it was needed. Share your feelings with your partner or friends, too.

"They told me I was going to have an emergency Cesarean and there wasn't time to wait for my husband to arrive. They didn't tell me what was happening, or if I'd be awake or asleep. I started shaking, just shaking. I couldn't stop. A doctor said to me, 'What's the matter?' and I said, 'I think I'm terrified.'"

If a woman is told why a procedure is needed by someone she has grown to trust, it becomes much easier to accept. This is true even about situations she had been strongly against:

"The midwife explained that if I didn't have an episiotomy, she thought I would have a bad tear. So I agreed to go ahead."

The woman in labor and her caregivers can often reach a compromise that satisfies them both. This mother felt she was still in control of her labor. And the doctors felt their advice was being respected: *"I think they are open to compromise also. I asked for more time in the second stage. I wanted to see if the contractions would sort themselves out and get started again. They said, 'OK, let's wait another twenty minutes.' I thought, "That's very sensible.""*

So don't be afraid to ask. Feeling happy after the birth is as important as being physically well.

Coping with Pain after a Cesarean

During the first 48 hours you will be offered a range of pain relief, which may include:

- Shots (given in your bottom or thigh) of pethidine or a similar drug for pain relief. (These drugs are safe to take if you are breast-feeding. Only a small amount passes to your baby in your milk.)

or

- Epidural top-ups, if you have had your Cesarean with an epidural

or

- A pump filled with a drug for pain relief attached to an IV drip in your arm. You work the pump yourself so that you can control your own pain relief. This is called *Patient-Controlled Analgesia* or *PCA*.

After 48 hours you will probably change to:

- Pain-killing tablets such as Tylenol®

THE IMPORTANT POINT IS:

Don't be afraid to ask for more pain-killers if you want them. Don't let pain prevent you from cuddling and feeding your baby.

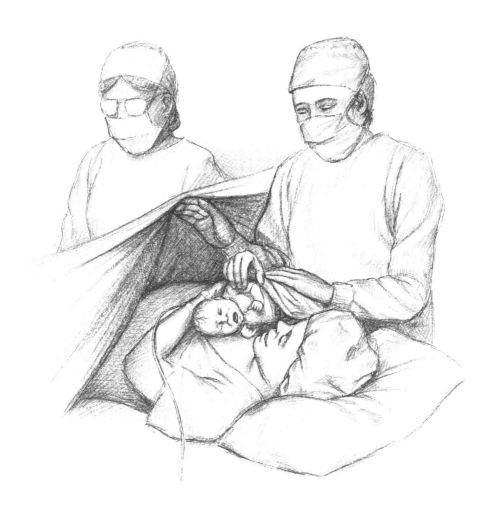

Taking Care of Yourself after a Cesarean

Getting out of bed

Curl your body so both knees come up to your chest. Then roll into a sitting position at the edge of the bed so you can get out. Nurses will help you.

Sitting in bed or in a chair

Use pillows for greater comfort. They help a lot when you are feeding your baby. Use the bell or buzzer to call for help if it is hard for you to lift your baby out of the crib.

Protecting your incision

Support your incision with a pillow or your hands when you cough, sneeze or laugh.

Coping with gas

Many women say the worst part of a Cesarean is the gas you suffer from afterward. The sooner you start walking, and the more you walk around, the fewer gas pains you will suffer.

Underwear

High-waisted panties feel best because they keep the pressure off your incision. You could also try men's boxer shorts.

Shoes

Slip-on slippers are the easiest. It may be hard to bend down to tie laces.

When home

Keep diaper things near you. Let the baby sleep close by, too. Then you won't have to go far to get to him.

Getting help

Line up help for when you get home—friends, family, anyone. Get your visitors working! Ask guests to make coffee, help with laundry and so on. Try not to do lifting or driving. It is best not to drive for up to four weeks after the operation.

Cascade of Intervention

Sometimes one intervention in labor leads to another. This chart suggests one possible sequence of events:

Midwife breaks the waters to speed up labor

Mother is monitored to see that her baby is coping without the bag of waters to buffer him from the contractions

Labor feels stronger and more painful now that the waters have gone and she cannot move around

She asks for an epidural

The epidural prevents her from pushing well during the second stage of labor

The baby becomes exhausted because of the length of second stage

A forceps birth is performed

Mother has a lot of stitches, which make it hard for her to sit to breastfeed her baby

Learning how to breastfeed is harder than it might have been otherwise.

Each intervention in labor carries risks as well as benefits. There are few real emergencies in childbirth. There is almost always time to consult with your caregivers about what to do next. Often, there are a few options to choose from. You and your doctor or midwife may decide on an intervention. Or you may decide otherwise.

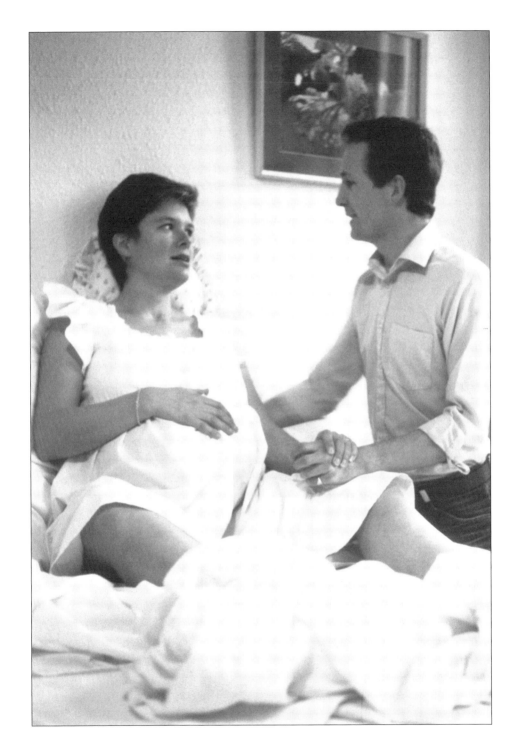

CHAPTER 7 *Labor Support*

No two labors are the same. If you have had a baby already, what happened during your first labor is not guaranteed to repeat itself next time. But your labors may be similar. If you're about to go through your first labor, you cannot know how things might go. "Not knowing" accounts for a large part of the nervousness women facing labor feel.

Think back to childhood. When you faced some difficult task, did you sometimes bring along your best friend? Having someone's hand to hold, to support you and be on your side, helped you find the courage to face what you had to do. As adults, we often have to confront challenges on our own. We accept this as part of the process of growing up. But labor is one time when you can still choose to have someone with you. Choose someone who is part of your daily life, whom you know well and who is there just to support you. Whether you have your baby at home or in a hospital, labor support is likely to help you relax and increase your enjoyment of birth.

There has been a lot of research about labor support. The results have often been staggering. Labor support can alter the events of labor itself and also how the woman feels about her labor afterwards. Studies have shown that women with support during labor need fewer painkillers. They also receive fewer interventions. They give birth to stronger babies. And after their babies are born, women who had support in labor feel better about themselves, their labors and their babies!

Fathers

It used to be that a woman who was having a baby always had other women to support her—her mother, her sister, a friend or all of these. Birth was a time when women rallied around and gave each other support. It was felt women were best able to give labor support because of their natural rapport with a woman in labor. It was almost unheard

147

The Labor-Support Role

Research suggests that nothing is more helpful to a woman coping with labor than good support from her doctor or midwife and her chosen labor companion. Loving support reduces a woman's need for pain-killing drugs and interventions in labor. It also improves her feelings about the birth.

So how can you help?

• First, help the mother get comfortable during labor. If she wants to stand or kneel or sit or lie on her side, help her do so. Then help her change her position when she needs to. If she is kneeling, she might like a pillow under her knees and ankles. If she is sitting astride a chair, she might like a pillow across the back of the chair to lean on. If she is standing, she might want to lean against you. You might rock with her from side to side. She might want to squat down between your legs and lean against your thighs if you are sitting on a chair.

• A woman needs to be loved and touched during labor. She may push you away one moment, but she will almost certainly want a hug the next! Tell her she's wonderful. When labor gets tough, a woman may begin to feel she's not coping well. It helps her a lot to know that *you* value the effort she is making and believe in her.

• The mother may be trying to help herself through contractions by keeping her breathing even. If her shoulders become hunched and tense, her breathing may become panicky. You can help by leaning gently on her shoulders so they drop down and her breathing relaxes. She might like you to breathe through contractions with her. Keep eye contact with her and encourage her to copy you: Breathe in calmly through your nose and blow out gently through your mouth.

• Information is vital to help the mother relax (and to help you relax as well). A woman in labor needs to know her baby is OK. You can ask the doctor or nurse the questions the mother may not be able to ask herself. Then you can pass the information to her. She will hear and understand what you say better than what the doctor says.

of for a man to be with his wife during labor, even though almost all women gave birth at home. In many cultures in the world today, women remain the only witnesses of labor and birth.

When women started giving birth in hospitals, they lost their traditional sources of support. Hospitals did not want the women present who might once have offered their help to a friend or relative in labor. Hospitals were strictly for healthcare providers. Some labor support was given by the nurse or midwife. But she might have several women

What Is Useful for Labor Support

- *Drinks and snacks* (for you and the mother)—Sandwiches, nuts and raisins, fruit and chocolate, and juices. Don't bring strong-smelling or highly flavored foods. These might make the mother feel sick.

- *Frozen juice or ice cubes*—If you are going to a hospital, put the cubes in a wide-mouth thermos. They're wonderful for the mother to suck on between contractions. You may enjoy them too.

- *Socks and a warm shawl*—Toward the end of the first stage of labor, the mother may feel very cold. She may enjoy the comfort of a shawl around her shoulders or socks to warm her feet.

- *Unscented vegetable oil*—This may be used for massaging the mother's back or shoulders.

- *Soft face towel*—For you to give to the mother to wipe her face, neck and hands.

- *Small natural sponge*—This can be soaked in iced water for the mother to suck on between contractions. Or use it to wipe her face gently. A natural sponge has a much more pleasant texture than a synthetic one.

- *Tapes and cassette player, or CDs and CD player*—So you and the mother can listen to your favorite music to help you relax during labor. (Check with the hospital to make sure you are allowed to use a portable sound system.)

- *Camera and film*—To take lots of photos of the new baby!

- *Small change for the phone or a phone card (and your personal address book)*—So you can spread the good news after the birth of the baby!

under her care at once. She could not stay with just one person. Nor was she necessarily someone known to the woman in labor. In addition, the nurse or midwife had many tasks to perform, so she was generally perceived by the woman in labor as part of the hospital rather than as someone who was there entirely to support her.

During the 1970s, women's groups began to campaign for fathers to be allowed to stay with their partners during labor. Men started to insist on having greater participation in family life. And women have always needed good support during labor. As actively involved members of the family, more men began to assist at the births of their children. It was not easy to change the hospital system. Fathers had been barred from the delivery room for a long time. However, in time, the campaign was a great success. Today, fathers are *expected* to be present at the birth of their babies. Indeed, there may now be *too much* pressure on men to support their partners in labor. Some fathers feel they cannot assume this role. But a lot of men are glad to be present.

Those Who Provide Labor Support Need to Look after Themselves

• Labor wards can be cold. It's good to bring along a warm shirt or jacket, just in case. You may still get hot because you will be working hard to support the laboring woman. Think in terms of layers of clothing that you can put on or take off as you need to. Wear a T-shirt, open-necked shirt or loose clothes. If you become too hot, you will start to feel faint. It will not be helpful to the mother, the nurse or the midwife if you pass out!

• Just as the mother needs food in early labor and lots of drinks as labor progresses, so do you. There's no shame in having a snack if you need one. You will be better able to support the mother if you are not grouchy or weak from hunger.

• You might need a short time away from the mother now and then. It can be extremely stressful being with someone who is going through a traumatic and painful time. If you want to leave the room for a few minutes, do so. The nurse or midwife will care for the mother until you return. She may also come get you if necessary!

• You need to know and understand what is happening during the labor as much as the mother. Ask all the questions you want. Create a good relationship with the midwife. That way, she may consult you as well as the mother about decisions regarding management of the labor.

• After the baby is born, talk to someone about what happened during the labor, how you felt and how you feel now. Mothers need to debrief their labors. So do those who support them. Women who gave birth have an easier time finding people who will listen to them talk about their birth experience than do the people who gave them support. Men who provide labor support may have a hard time finding someone with whom to talk. Try and think of someone to whom you can turn.

Still, research suggests that most men do not take an active part in labor but are simply there as onlookers. This isn't hard to understand. A man who attends the birth of his child is entering a woman's world, perhaps for the first time. He may not fully understand the birth process. He may be frightened and distressed by his partner's pain. He may not like seeing her behave in ways she would not normally behave. He may be upset by the sight of blood. On top of this, he has to cope with the huge change in his own life that is taking place during labor. Just as his partner is becoming a mother, he is becoming a father. It is hard to support another person when your own emotions are in turmoil.

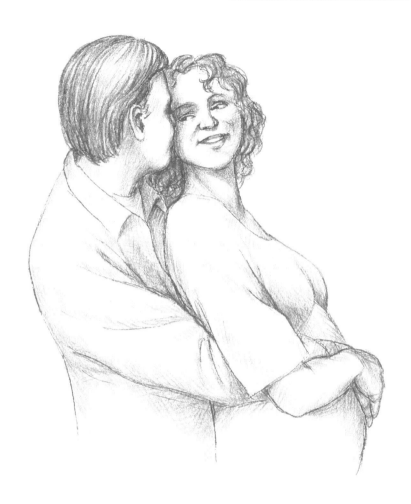

Despite this, many men seem to support their partners very well during labor, as these women confirm.

"It's someone you know very well, who can talk to you and take your mind off everything. He understood what I was hollering about."

"My husband was there. He did nothing at all except carry my bag and sit and watch. He didn't say anything to me, but he was very reassuring and very calm. Having him there just a few yards away made it all better. I think I would have coped less well if I'd been on my own even though, looking back, there's nothing much he did."

"It's important to have someone you love there."

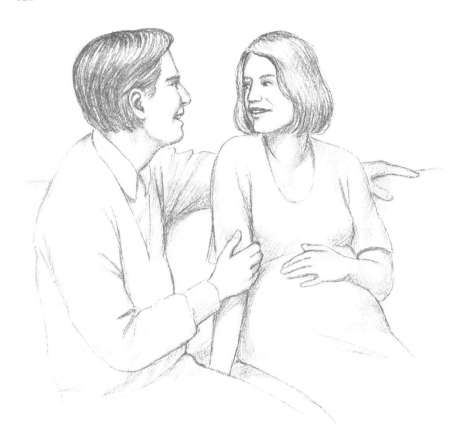

"I wouldn't want anyone else to see me in labor. I've got a friend who is a midwife. I wondered beforehand whether I would like her with me. I don't think I would because I wouldn't want her to see me like that. But I felt happy with John. I mean John has seen me at my worst. *I took it for granted he would be there. I wouldn't have wanted anyone else."*

Many women report an immediate effect on their labor if their partner left the room: *"When Brett went out, just for a minute, to go to the bathroom or something, the contractions got a lot worse because he wasn't there."*

When labor is complicated or a C-section is needed, a father can do nothing except be with the woman. But his presence at such times is even more important than during uncomplicated labor. *"Gilbert being there during the operation was really important. It was very frightening to go through that. He was a real support. He was telling me what was going on and he was just wonderful."*

Sometimes men are not allowed to stay in the room when medical procedures or internal exams are performed. This can distress the woman very much. You (or your partner) might want to be assertive and ask the reason for your partner being sent out. *"I don't understand why they sent Jim away when I was having my epidural. That was the time I needed him most. That was the time it was hurting the most. I was completely on my own. I panicked. At least if someone is with you, he can hold your hand and look at you and tell you everything's going to be all right."*

Men can do a number of helpful things if they are able to be more involved with the labor.

"He was very useful because he kept taking me to the bathroom. That was good because I felt scared about going on my own."

"He kept saying, 'You're doing really well; that's right, you're doing really well.'"

"My husband was a great support, rubbing my back, just firm pressure in the small of my back."

"Whenever I was on the verge of losing my grip, he'd say: 'Just concentrate, concentrate.'"

The father can also be an advocate for the woman. He can explain to the staff what she wants. *"Even when I'd been given Demerol, he was still being vocal about what we wanted to happen. He kept going to bat for me. He would say, 'Well, I don't think this is what we want to happen here,' or, 'Could you explain why you want to do that to her?' Although I was pretty out of it at this stage, he was still very much stating what our position was. He was very supportive."*

Some men are naturals at labor support. They seem to know just how to help. *"He would say, 'Get ready with your breathing, now,' because he could see the contraction building [on the monitor]. The two of us were really working together. It was incredible."*

When the father doesn't want to be there

Some men just do not want to be present at the birth of their baby. And some women feel that their partner would not be helpful. *"My partner*

missed the birth because they took me in to be induced and then it happened very quickly. But looking back on it, I'm glad he wasn't there.
He'd been with me when they gave me the Prostin® gel and he kept saying, 'I don't like this.' I think I dealt with the labor very well. But if I'd
had to think about him also, I'm not sure what would have happened.
They took blood from the baby's head at one stage, and that was traumatic enough for me. But if he'd been there watching, it would have
been awful. We both agree that what we want next time is for him to
come in just after the birth."

Birth is the outcome of the sexual act. It is itself sexual and involves
the most intimate parts of the woman's body. For some men, seeing
their partner exposed to the gaze of a nurse (possibly a male nurse)
and perhaps of male doctors, is profoundly upsetting. Viewing their
partner's pain and perhaps seeing the woman's sexual organs damaged
during birth can give rise to feelings of guilt. Such feelings may have a
long-term effect on the couple's sex lives.

*"Steve doesn't want to be present for the birth, and I agree. The last birth
had dramatic effects on our sex life. We had no sex life at all for a long
time after the birth. I think part of it was that he watched me and saw
me doing things I don't normally do and behaving in a way I don't normally behave. And he saw me being snipped and stitched. It was a lot
for him to have watched. I think it made him feel helpless. He couldn't
do anything to help. He felt if he hadn't had sex with me, I wouldn't
have been going through that."*

It is almost certain not to be helpful if a man agrees to be present
during labor when he really doesn't want to be. Whether he will be
present is a mutual decision. And it's still possible—even with today's
pressures—for a couple to decide that the father will *not* be present.
He can often be helping out elsewhere in the family. *"We've agreed
that because he doesn't really feel the need to be there, he'll look after
our little girl while I'm having the baby."*

The experience of fathers

A man's experience of pregnancy, labor and early parenthood mirrors
the woman's. It often consists of a great deal of worry, as well as pride
and excitement. Although his life is also going through a radical
change, he may receive much less support than she does. Others may
be much less aware that something major is happening to him. When

fathers talk about labor, it is clear they ride on the same emotional roller-coaster as their partners do. The time spent waiting for labor to start can be highly charged.

"She started having very mild contractions. I couldn't sleep because I didn't want to miss anything. Then the contractions stopped. There were a few days of 'Is she or isn't she?,' which was completely exhausting."

"Waiting for labor was almost unbearable."

When labor finally starts, the father's feelings are likely to be the same as the mother's. *"I felt a mixture of relief that the labor had started and terror at what was going to happen."*

Many men enjoy having a part to play during the labor. Doing something distracts from the worry about whether the labor is going well. It also helps fathers cope with their partner's pain.

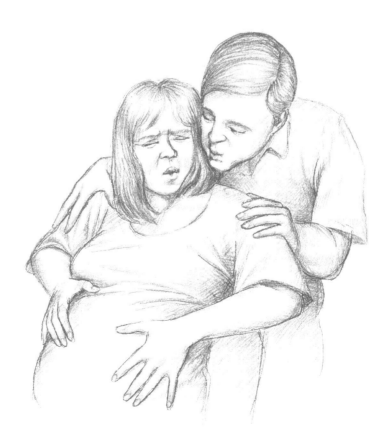

Checklist for Labor Support: PURRRR

Position

Is the mother changing her position often and moving around?

Urination

Are you reminding her to go to the bathroom every hour?

Relaxation

Is she as relaxed as possible?

Respiration

Is she breathing evenly and not gasping?

Rest

Is she making the most of the break between contractions to rest and refresh herself?

Reassurance

Are you giving her constant encouragement and reassurance?

"I did some back massage to help her through the contractions. I wanted to be involved. I wanted to be needed—and loved—as well."

But often, a father may feel there is nothing he can do. And while the woman is totally focused on her contractions, he is left to cope with the intensity of his own emotions, as these three men describe:

"For the last few hours of Monica's labor, I was horrified by the amount of pain she was going through."

"At times I was physically sick from worry."

"All I could do during the really tough parts was talk, swallow hard and admire her courage as she pushed out the baby."

Guilt that they are partly the cause of the woman's suffering is often on fathers' minds: *"When I remember what Janet went through, I feel uneasy talking about the birth."*

Some men do not look back on their presence at their partner's labor with any pleasure. *"To be honest, it was probably one of the most unpleasant events of my life."*

The moment of birth can be overwhelming. Fathers can match the intensity of the mother's emotions in combining joy at the birth of the baby with relief that labor is safely over, as these two new fathers describe:

"I cried and cried and my whole body ached. I was so relieved that the baby was absolutely fine and that Hannah was absolutely fine."

"Before the birth, I never thought about holding him. The nurse gave him to me and he was so alive—looking at me—and so innocent."

Doulas

Doula is a Greek word. A doula is a woman who has given birth herself and has reared children. Her job is to help other women give birth and to teach them how to care for their babies.

How doulas help women in labor—What the research shows

In the 1980s, three doctors working in the large maternity hospital in Guatemala City wanted to see whether women would have shorter labors if they had someone to support them. At the time, women in labor at this hospital were not allowed to have companions with them during labor. They were left on their own by the midwives until just before their babies were born. Their labors tended to be very long.

The doctors recruited women who were mothers themselves to come into the hospital as labor supporters or *doulas*. The doulas were instructed to do nothing more than hold the woman who was in labor, talk to her, massage her, encourage her and stay with her until her baby was born. By taking this simple step, the average length of labor was reduced for women having their first babies from 19 hours to 8 hours! Women who had doulas were far less likely to need a Cesarean section or forceps than women who had no one to support them. They also gave birth to healthier babies. Since this famous study was carried out, it has been shown that, not just in third-world countries, but also in affluent Western countries, women still have fewer complications in labor and healthier babies if they are supported by a doula. After the birth, women who have had doula support tend to feel good about their labors. They also tend to

form a close bond with their babies very quickly. It appears that being "mothered" while in labor helps a woman become a satisfied mother herself.

Why can't midwives be doulas?

Many midwives would like to be doulas. They see their role as supporting the woman in labor by responding to her physical and emotional needs. However, midwives are often very busy people, even if they are only caring for one woman. In many hospitals, each midwife will have several women in labor under her care. This "busy-ness" may prevent the midwife from simply staying close to the mother. A midwife may not have the time to hold and comfort her, to notice her changes of mood, or to offer the small physical comforts that make labor easier. It is more likely for a midwife to offer the kind of support a doula offers if the mother is giving birth at home. But even then she has to make sure that certain procedures are carried out at certain times and that records are kept carefully. That divides her attention to some extent.

Would it cost too much to hire a doula?

Marsden Wagner of the World Health Organization (WHO) figures the United States could save a billion dollars a year if doulas were employed to support women in labor. This figure is based on research that has shown far fewer women have forceps or ventouse (vacuum) births or Cesarean sections when they are supported by doulas. Fewer of their babies need to be cared for in neonatal intensive care units (NICUs).

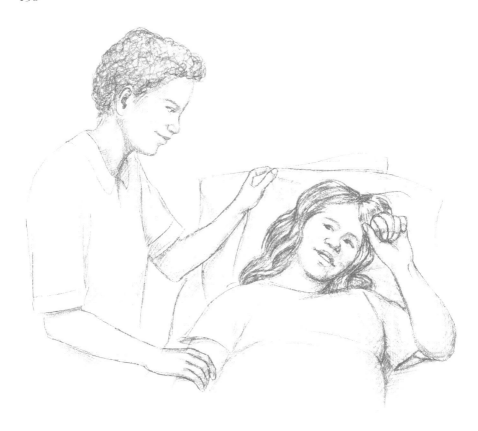

Other Labor Support

Some women choose to have both their partner and a woman support them in labor. There is good research to show how effective support from a woman can be in improving the outcome of labor. Female labor support can also help a new mother feel confident about taking on the duties of caring for her new baby. In some areas, a pregnant woman can hire a doula, a woman trained to provide labor support. The two get to know each other during the last weeks of pregnancy. The doula then supports the mother through labor and visits her in the hospital or at home afterward. The doula helps a new mother with baby-care tasks. She also helps her adjust to the emotions of becoming a parent.

Most of the time, though, if a mother chooses to have a woman with her to provide labor support, it is a relative or a good friend.

"I'd like my sister or a very close friend to be there too. It gives your partner a break. They can take turns looking after you. Also, having another woman there is different from having a man there. Maybe she can empathize better with what's going on."

"My instinctive feeling is to have women around me. I'll ask a friend to stay in the house to look after me."

One choice for some women is their mother, if you get along well. *"My mom was wonderful. She has this positive vibe about her that communicates, 'You can do it. Let's do it right.' Maybe it's because she's been through it herself, but she really made a difference. She made good, practical suggestions and was just so positive."*

"During the actual birth, Darryl was there. That was very comforting, but it was my sister I hung onto. I tried to lean on Darryl, but he was too tall and I couldn't get comfortable. She was just the right height and it was a lot easier."

At home, you can choose to have whoever you want present for the birth. Most hospitals are fairly flexible, although some may prefer you to have just one person. Think carefully about who will be with you. The person or people whom you choose to provide labor support will certainly affect how you feel about your labor afterward. They may also influence what happens during it. If you already have children, you might want to consider whether you want them to be present at the birth. *"My 3-year-old daughter was with me during most of the labor. It felt right for her to be there."*

Adults often worry that small children will be upset if they see their mother in pain. They worry that children will be frightened by the sounds she makes and the sight of blood. But research suggests children take it all in stride. Some studies have found that children who are present at the birth of a sibling have a special closeness with him or her. Women who choose to have their children with them are showing that birth is, for them, a family affair: *"Robbie was cuddling me between contractions. He was very supportive and not bothered by my contractions at all. When the baby was being born, he stroked my shoulder. And when the baby's head came out, he said, 'Baby . . . baby.' When she was born, I was crying but he knew somehow that I wasn't sad. I think the fact that he was there helped us bond as a family."*

Support from Nurses and Midwives

Labor nurses and midwives are special people who come into your life for a short time but can make a profound impact on it. It is essential to get along with the nurse who cares for you in labor. You need to feel you can trust her advice and know she will not do anything without taking your opinion and feelings into account first. Women often see a different doctor or midwife at each clinic visit. They walk into the delivery suite at the hospital not knowing who is going to look after them. The result of meeting different providers at each prenatal visit, and of seeing more doctors and nurses during and after the birth can be negative: *"I saw about eight different nurses in the hospital and different doctors, too. To me, it was really confusing. They were each telling me to do different things. After the birth it was even worse."*

Many health plans these days enable women to get to know just a small group of doctors or midwives who provide all their care. Sometimes you can even choose to be cared for by a certain doctor or midwife. You can always ask if such a scheme is part of your health plan, as these three women did:

"I have the same midwife this time that I had for my last labor. She was the one I wanted. We've looked at my notes and talked about what I want."

"I asked for one certain midwife. I'm nervous anyway and I want the chance to get to know her. Although a birth plan is nice if you've never been pregnant before, it can be kind of unreal. It's fine to write things down but you don't know what labor's going to be like when it happens. I've talked through my feelings about it with the midwife."

"I think if I hadn't had the midwife I knew, my birth might not have gone so well. She respected my views because of the trust that we had built between us."

Women explain how the best nurses and midwives are the ones who believe in you. They offer both physical and emotional support. They always keep you informed and respect your opinions. And they clearly care about you and want what is best for you.

"My labor nurse was super. She never, ever gave out any negative vibes. She was always positive."

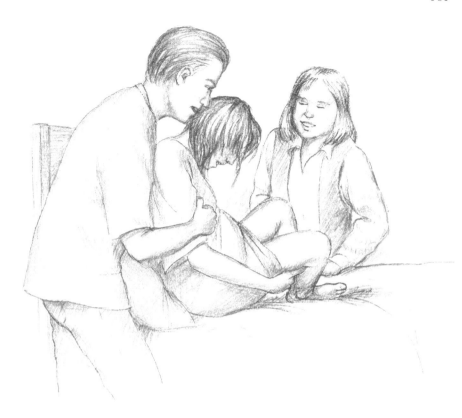

"A midwife popped into the room. She was a wonderful lady who literally hugged me. She was the best physical support I had. She was wonderful. She was a big-busted lady with a bright red T-shirt. I was literally hugged while I was pushing and it was wonderful."

"The nurse was supportive and reassuring. She let me know what was going on."

"I was glad the nurse who'd been with me in labor came along when I went to have a Cesarean. It helped to see a familiar face."

"The midwives—you couldn't fault them. They consulted me. They asked me what I wanted. They explained everything."

"The nurses came to see me in my room afterward, which was so nice. They took an interest. They really cared."

If a woman is unsure about how her partner will cope during labor, she may be relieved to know the labor nurse will try to look after him as well as her. *"I know my husband will feel better if everything isn't left up to him. He's pretty tough but he'll still feel a little upset and anxious at seeing me in pain. He'll be glad if the nurse is behind him telling him what to do."*

Midwives don't have to take over from others who provide labor support. They can simply show the supporters how to be helpful to the woman. *"She advised Tom to do back massage, which really helped. It was wonderful to have someone there to help us both through it."*

Not having a nurse in whom she feels confidence has the same effect on a woman as sensing that her partner doesn't really want to be with her in labor. She becomes more and more anxious. Labor becomes more difficult. Nurses do not always provide the best sort of care to every woman. They may feel uneasy about the way a woman wants to handle labor. Or they may work in a place where they themselves do not receive adequate support.

"The next couple of hours are blurry. At eight o'clock the nurse-midwife suggested I try a shot of Demerol. I'm not sure why because I didn't want it. But I didn't question her. I think I didn't question her because I was aware that the midwife wasn't very relaxed. I didn't want to do anything to make her worse. I tried to crack jokes between contractions just to improve the atmosphere. I think she wanted me to be a 'good patient.' And I wanted to be able to relax and be just a woman in labor."

"Not all nurse-midwives are sensitive. In the second stage, she was saying to me, 'Breathe! Breathe!' I was obviously breathing. I was making a lot of noise and was coping really well. Later, when she was stitching me up, I said I was going to shout. As soon as I made a sound, the nurse-midwife backed off. She couldn't handle the noise at all. She couldn't deal with women using noise to cope with pain."

It's awful if a woman perceives that her nurse or labor-support person doubts she can give birth. A major theme that runs through women's accounts of their support in labor is whether their nurse or labor partner did or did not believe in them. *"At one point, the nurse whispered to a doctor who was passing in the corridor, 'Yes, she's pushing but she can't make it.' I thought, 'Oh God: I'm going to have a Cesarean.' To know the nurse and my husband were saying 'She can't do it' was a desperate moment. It was so stressful. That's when I was ready to*

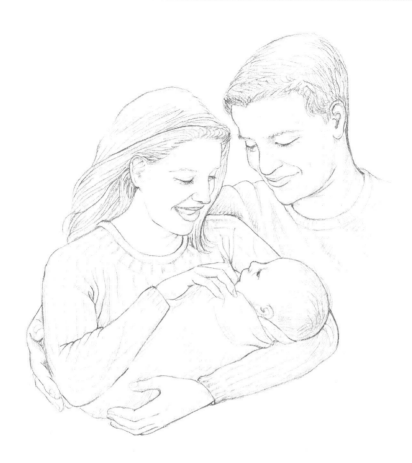

give up. You may appear *to be almost unconscious or in another world. But you're still sensitive to the little signals that show people are losing heart."*

When the woman's caregivers believe in her and show it, even a woman who is terrified of giving birth can be powered through her labor. *"My midwife kept telling me I could do it. I kept saying I couldn't do it, I couldn't cope. She kept saying, 'You* are *coping, you* are *doing it.' I kept asking for every form of pain relief I'd ever heard of. And she kept saying, 'No, you can do it without. And I did! She was right. I had no confidence I could do it, and she helped me a lot."*

Such caregivers do more for a woman than help her achieve a successful birth. They can influence how she feels about herself for the rest of her life. Caregivers can transmit their own confidence to the laboring woman so that she takes on her new role as a mother feeling on top of the world.

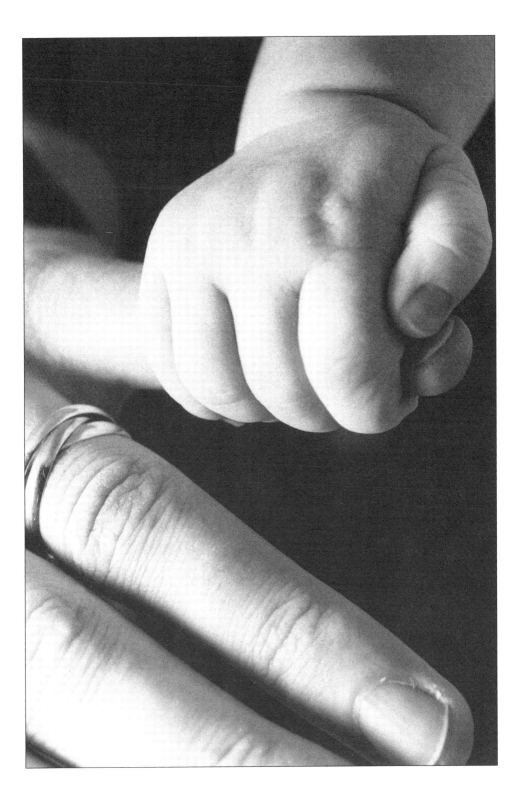

CHAPTER 8 *Fears and Losses*

There are all sorts of fears and losses involved in becoming pregnant and giving birth. When you are pregnant, you may have to change your daily routine. You might have to cope with feeling tired and sick. And you'll have to make time for prenatal checkups. Your old way of looking at the world changes. Some things move into sharper focus. Items on the news about people starving or about children suffering are suddenly charged with far stronger emotions than they were before. Pregnancy is a time when women often feel glowing and positive. But it's also a time of anxious thoughts. Will the baby be healthy? What will labor be like? And how will I cope afterward?

As the months pass, most women become more aware that the freedom they once enjoyed as a single person or as a couple will disappear when the baby is born. During labor, the birth plans they had made when they were pregnant are replaced by the events that really happen. When the baby is born, the baby of their pregnant dreams changes into a real baby. It has its own appearance and behavior. After the birth, their image of themselves as firm-bodied women changes. It is replaced by a body image that includes a round tummy and larger and softer breasts.

Fears about Not Coping with Labor Pain

Some women feel that they should not have to suffer while they are giving birth. Doctors have all sorts of pain-relief methods for use in labor. But a large number of women would prefer to manage without drugs or IV drips. They want to give their children a drug-free start. Labor is seen as a major hurdle in life: If you can leap it on your own, you have done something worthwhile. Women often feel that giving birth without medical help says something about their strength as a woman. This strong sense of wanting to cope with pain in labor on your own often runs beside a fear that it might not be possible:

"I'll try it for as long as I can. Then, if I feel I need some help, I'll ask for it. If I don't do it myself, I hope I won't feel like I've failed."

"You don't want to feel like you've failed. But if things go wrong, how can you be sure you won't feel that way?"

"I'm scared I'm going to give in and ask for an epidural. I really don't want to have an epidural."

Loss of the Labor You Wanted

Because there is no blueprint for labor, you can't predict what will happen. How a woman copes with pain in labor depends on so many things. How good is her support from her labor partner and doctor? What is her personal pain threshold? What is the place like in which she is giving birth? What position is her baby in inside her? How long is her labor? Are there any complications? And so on . . . Whatever happens, the woman will have very certain feelings about her labor after it is over. Giving birth is the kind of event you never forget:

"The first labor was great. It was just what you dream of, and I felt wonderful. But the birth of my second baby was nothing like the first one. The labor was half the length of the first, but very painful. I was so tired for days afterward. I was sad not to feel as great as I had the first time around. The second time, the baby was posterior. He looked squashed, and he came out angry. I was upset about the pain. I couldn't cope the way I'd coped the first time."

A woman who feels low after childbirth because the labor was not the way she would have liked it may not find much support: *"A lot of people say to me, 'But you've got a healthy baby! Why are you worried? Everything turned out all right.' But I can't get over how angry and mauled I feel because of what that went wrong in my labor. I didn't get along with the nurse who was with me. That was a let-down in itself. I think I could have had a very different birth if I'd had someone I really trusted."*

A Cesarean section may be life-saving for both mother and baby. But even when the woman knows there is a real need for her baby to be born this way, her feelings about it aren't always logical:

"When I think about loss, I think about my second birth. My first birth was so positive, at home. It was really amazing, and so nice. So I was shocked when, the next time, I ended up having an emergency Cesarean in the middle of the night. I had a hard band on one side of my cervix. It was caused by laser surgery I'd had between the two babies. Because of it, I couldn't dilate beyond 2cm. I felt I'd been robbed of my birth. It really upsets me to think I might never be able to have a vaginal birth again."

Not knowing what happened during the labor can cause women to feel unhappy about their births for years: *"I feel down about the Cesarean sometimes, and I have 'I don't care' phases also. At the moment, I wonder whether the Cesarean was really needed. I've been finding out more about what happened. I keep thinking, 'If only they'd left me another ten minutes . . . if only . . .' Jessie's two-and-a-half now and the sadness still comes in phases."*

Loss of control sums up labor for some women. They may have been overwhelmed with pain and didn't behave as they would have liked. Or perhaps they needed a large number of medical interventions to ensure a safe outcome: *"You feel cheated that it didn't happen the right way, the way you planned it."*

Meeting a Different Baby

You often imagine, while you are pregnant, what your baby will look like. The thoughts a woman has when she sees her baby for the first time become a vital part of her life. Pregnant women often look forward to that moment of meeting with great pleasure: *"I used to dream that he came out in the night. We had a look at him, and he wasn't quite ready, so we put him back! I had that dream a couple of times because I wanted to know what he looked like."*

"You can have very funny dreams where the baby has your face or your husband's face or an animal's face sometimes!"

When the new baby arrives, he or she may look nothing like the image you had in your mind:

"I turned over to look at her and saw the fattest baby I had ever seen. She looked like a cross between a Pekinese puppy and a Sumo wrestler."

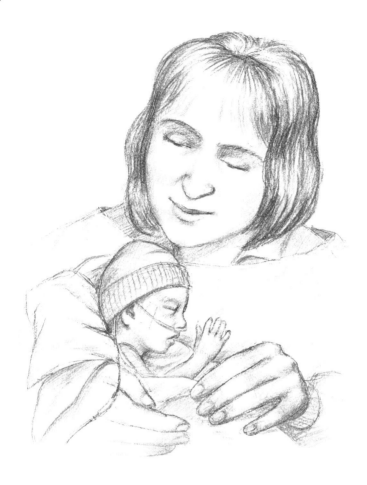

"Who was this bluish, squinting, skinny thing?"

"I looked down and thought, 'Oh my God! It's got purple skin and green hair.' I was so shocked. He'd moved his bowels as he was being born. Sludge was all over him. He had a lot of hair, and he came out with green hair!"

The baby may not be the sex the mother had wanted. Women often find it hard to express their feelings about this. Many cultures find it wrong to grieve over a baby who is perfectly well but not of the desired sex:

"I really wanted a girl the third time around because I already had two boys. I was really upset to have another boy. I'm not going to have any more children. So I'll never have a little girl now."

Not Meeting the Baby

Some women who have had long, hard labors are in no shape to greet their babies when they are born: *"I can vaguely remember trying to hold this slippery bundle. I tried to unravel the cord that was around her. I can't remember what she looked like, and that makes me really sad. It must be because of the drugs. They took her away, and I fell back onto some cushions. I didn't even think about where she was."*

The emotions you feel at birth may not be what you had expected: *"Every mom would like to feel this great love when she first meets her baby. But it doesn't always work that way. I felt nothing for my baby— just vaguely anxious because she looked so blue. I said, 'Give her to my husband.'"*

A mother who gives birth to twins may find that she is so caught up with the baby who has been born first that she misses the moment when the second is born: *"It scared me that she didn't cry and she was purple. She was whisked away to get help with her breathing. I forgot about the other twin completely, I was so worried about Carrie. I didn't even know when our little boy was born."*

Mothers whose babies need special care may also miss the joy of seeing and holding their babies as soon as they are born: *"I had her at 9:05 in the morning. I didn't even wake up until eleven. Then they said, 'It's a girl and she's all right.' But I was so drugged, I couldn't go see her. I kept saying, 'Can I go see her yet, can I go and see her yet?' But they wouldn't let me. They did show me her photo, which helped. And Mark kept rushing off to intensive care. But it was very hard not being able to see her for over 12 hours."*

"She had blue eyes, although she was very gray-looking. I held her for a moment. Her eyes were really striking. Then she was rushed off to intensive care. I kept thinking, 'I want to see my baby! Where's my baby?' I felt that precious hours were being lost when I should have been with my baby."

It can be a great shock to expect to have a gorgeous, healthy baby, and instead give birth to a small, sick one: *"Because I am a big person, I thought I was going to have this great big baby. Instead I had this tiny baby that was being tube-fed. I couldn't even hold him. And I didn't see him on the day I had him . . . I can't explain what that did to me."*

Sickly babies can seem like complete strangers to their parents: *"My partner and I were taken to see the twins in the intensive-care unit. We touched their tiny hands and cried because they were so small. Then we went back to the ward. We felt like we didn't know our babies at all."*

Women who go to the hospital to give birth look forward to the day they will bring their babies home to meet their families. But mothers whose babies need long-term special care have to come home on their own: *"I was OK while I was in the hospital. But when I came home and he was still in there, that was hard. When I came home after the last visit of the day, I'd cry all night. It was so hard to leave him there."*

The Death of a Baby

Sometimes birth and death come close together. The event, which was expected to bring with it so much happiness, turns into a tragedy. When this happens, parents suffer an intense let-down:

"The baby was very still and there was no sound."

"My baby was found to be dead at 38 weeks. Her heartbeat had been heard clearly at 37 weeks. We went home and came back to induce labor the next day. When she was born, the midwife took her right out of the room. We had said we didn't want to see her. Then she came and asked if we were sure about that. We told her we would like to see her after all. As soon as we looked at her, we called her Sarah. We knew then that we had lost a member of our family."

Soon after the first shock comes the rush of questions: *"Why us? Why did it have to happen? What did I do wrong?"*

Most hospitals are far better at caring for grieving parents than they used to be. Parents are given time to hold their baby for as long as they want. If they don't meet their baby, it's very hard to grieve for a person they have never known. When the mother dresses her dead baby in his own clothes and cuddles him and weeps over him, she knows that this baby was a real little person who was alive and is now dead. Parents are encouraged to take pictures of their baby. They can be given a hand print or footprint and a lock of the baby's hair. Most hospitals now have a special Book of Remembrance. Grieving parents can write the name of their miscarried or stillborn baby in it, and a few words about him. Some parents find that they cannot do this right away. But they return to the hospital, perhaps many months later, to put their baby's name in the book.

While parents are feeling numb, funeral plans have to be made. Friends and family tend to rally around. But once the funeral is over, bereaved parents can feel very much alone. People often find it hard to cope with the death of a baby. Many don't know what to say to the parents. They sometimes make hurtful comments simply because they are so distressed themselves: *"'You're young. You can have another baby.' It was like saying, 'Your best friend has died. But don't worry, you can get a new one.'"*

Nature can also seem cruel at this time. Despite the fact the baby is dead, the mother's breasts still make the milk that would have been needed had he lived: *"For the first three weeks, my sore breasts were a constant reminder of our loss."*

After the first period of intense grieving, parents often find they need to talk about their feelings and their baby:

"Talk, talk, talk is the best therapy."

"I was very lucky. A number of friends let me talk about Bradley. They didn't get embarrassed if I cried. Sometimes they cried too. Talking was my best medicine."

Women may need to talk to their doctor or midwife about their pregnancy to find out why things went wrong. The healthcare provider can often explain that nothing she did or did not do had any effect on the outcome of her pregnancy. But healthcare providers cannot always explain why her baby died. The mother and her partner still need to have the chance to talk to a healthcare provider. They will find comfort in knowing they are fully informed.

The best people to talk to are those who have also lost a baby and *really know* how you feel. Their support is special: *"I found it hard to talk to my mother or to close family. I knew they were suffering as well, and I didn't want to distress them any more. I had a friend who lost her baby about six weeks before me. Talking to her helped a lot."*

Bereaved parents can contact groups such as Sidelines or SHARE. Sidelines is a nonprofit group that puts women in touch with volunteers who have gone through similar troubles. SHARE is a support-group organization, with chapters across North America (see Appendix).

"I had to talk to people who had had a similar tragedy. They understood the powerful emotions I was going through."

Not Pregnant Any More

Despite all the discomforts and worries of pregnancy, many women really enjoy those nine months. They like being the center of attention and feel proud and special. No matter how happy the mother is when her baby is born, she can still feel regretful that she isn't pregnant any more:

"I really felt the loss of my belly when I had the baby. I enjoyed people getting out of my way and helping me across the street."

"I loved my stomach from the very first moment I knew I was pregnant. I sang to my stomach in the shower. I used to rub it. Not having my big stomach any more makes me feel very sad."

"I felt great when I was pregnant. I was never alone. If I was frightened, I used to sit and talk to the baby inside me. It comforted me."

After the birth, attention tends to shift away from the woman and onto her baby. For the mother, it can be hard to carry the baby for nine months, go through labor and then find that she seems less important:

"When you are pregnant, people make a fuss over you. The minute you have the baby, you come in second. You never get the same attention again. They want to see the baby. They'll ask how you are, but it's the baby they really care about. That's a real shock to the system."

Loss of Independence

It's hard to imagine while you are still pregnant just how demanding a new baby can be. No one would believe how many hours of the day and night are needed to keep up with feeding and diaper changing and soothing. We often find becoming a mother difficult because we have so many other things that we need or want to do. There just doesn't seem to be enough time for everything. You can feel an enormous frustration when the routine you used to enjoy is turned upside down. Women are perfectly aware when they're pregnant that life will change after the birth of their babies. But just how big that change will be is hard to anticipate. *"What I'm frightened of is a loss of energy. I just*

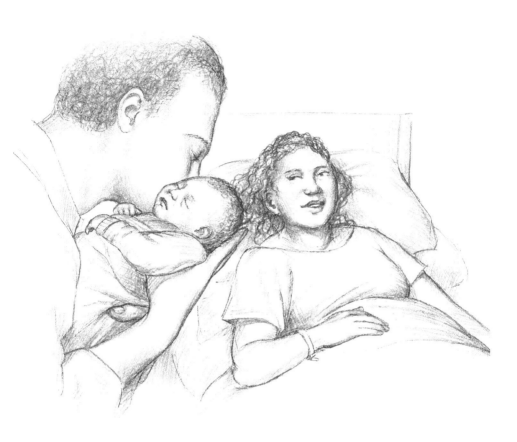

think I won't have any energy. I might not feel well, and I won't be able
to do anything. I'm worried about that. I also worry about my loss of
independence. People keep telling me that my life is never going to be
the same again. So I worry about the loss of me as the person I now am."*

After the baby is born, the freedom you once enjoyed is replaced by
a burden, which can sometimes seem very heavy. You must provide
completely for someone else's well-being:

*"My baby was so very, very little. He was so dependent on me. That was
really scary."*

*"You know the buck stops with you. You can call your mother and
everything, but in the end, the buck stops with you. That's frightening."*

The burden can feel heavier when the mother is extremely tired. The loss of peaceful sleep is a very real one: *"I miss my sleep. That's a real sense of loss."*

Getting Help

It's normal to have a sense of loss as well as happiness after your baby is born. It takes time to settle into a new role as a mother. Your body will also take some weeks to recover from labor. Your emotions will take at least as long and maybe much longer to calm down. It often helps to talk about your labor and how you feel about your new baby to someone else who listens well. Some women find it helpful to write down the events of their birth and keep a journal of the first weeks of motherhood. Putting their feelings on paper helps them to understand: *"I wrote it all down and it made sense. I think it's one of the things that helped me."*

Some hospitals make sure that each woman has a chance to debrief (review) her labor. If you have your baby at home, your doctor or midwife may give you the chance to talk about what happened the next time they visit. It helps to go over the events of your labor with the doctor or midwife who cared for you when your baby was born. Then she can explain why things happened the way they did. She can make sure the questions that might cause you concern in the future are answered. Many women feel that: *"All hospitals should provide a debriefing service. Otherwise we carry these events with us forever."*

The best form of support after you become a mother is likely to be other women who are also mothers. Seek them out if your circle of friends doesn't include women with babies. Other mothers of tiny babies *know* how you are feeling. Without doubt, they are the people who are best able to offer you sound, practical advice and support.

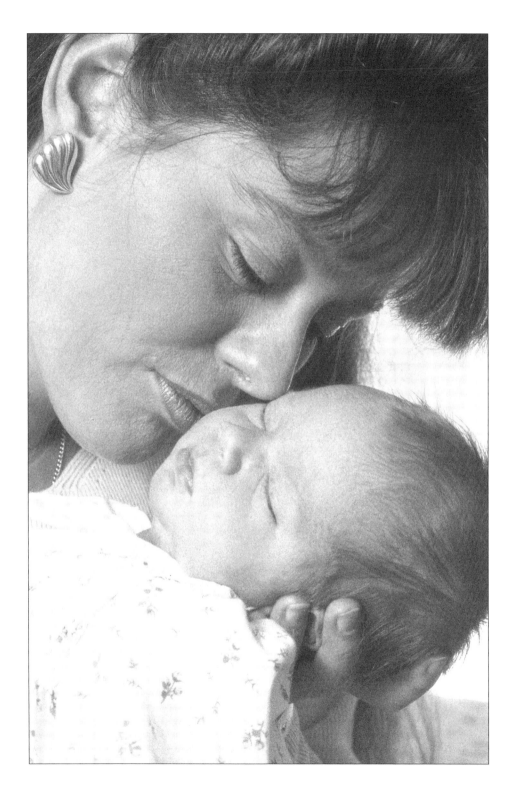

CHAPTER 9 *The First Days*

The first few hours and days after the birth of your baby are filled with changes in your body and in your emotions. Your body is suddenly no longer pregnant. It goes through huge changes as the uterus shrinks in size and starts to return to its nonpregnant state.

All the fluid that gathered in your body while you were pregnant has to be eliminated. Women who have just given birth may find they need to go to the toilet often—as frequently as they did at the end of their pregnancies.

The breasts respond to hormones that instruct them to make colostrum and then mature milk. If you decide not to breast-feed your baby, the breasts have to respond to the fact that the baby is not being put to the breast and no milk is required.

With all that is going on inside your body, many women feel mentally exhausted after labor, or a few days later. Friends and family react to the news that the baby has been safely born with delight. The news is "so wonderful" and the parents should feel "insane with joy."

Mothers often find their emotions are turbulent during the first days after the birth. They have times when they feel extremely happy and times when they feel extremely sad. A joyous birth may turn into a bout of crying and despair when the baby blues set in a few days later.

Women can find themselves trying to look like a pleased and caring mother while feeling very insecure. They can feel very much aware of the heavy burden of the baby. And they often feel resentful of the loss of their personal space.

Checking Your Baby at Birth

The Doctor or Midwife's Exam

Within the first hour of your baby's birth, the doctor or midwife will look him over carefully. She needs to make sure he is healthy. She will check:

- *His eyes:* to see if they are a normal distance apart and that each lens is clear.

- *His mouth:* to make sure the hard palate is complete (not cleft) and that the baby has no teeth. (Sometimes a baby is born with a few teeth. These are often loose and need to be taken out in case the baby breathes them into his lungs.)

- *His breathing:* to see that he is breathing through his nose and not through his mouth.

- *His head:* to check the shape of the skull and that the soft spots on the baby's head are normal.

- *His chest and abdomen:* to check that the breathing movements of the baby's chest are regular and that his abdomen is round.

- *The stump of the umbilical cord:* to check that there are three blood vessels. (The doctor or nurse will probably remove the metal forceps that were clipped onto the cord when your baby was born. She will replace them with a plastic clamp.)

- *The genitals:* to make sure that the penis is open at the end. A girl baby is checked to make sure she has two openings, one from her vagina and one from her urethra.

- *The back passage (rectum):* to make sure it is open. (The doctor or nurse will take the baby's temperature by putting a thermometer gently into his back passage. This is the most precise way of finding a baby's temperature.)

- *His spine:* to make sure the backbone has formed properly.

- *His hands and feet:* to make sure there are ten fingers and ten toes! They also check that the baby can move his wrists and ankles normally.

The doctor or midwife will measure around the baby's head and his length from the top of his head to his heels. She will also weigh him.

The Pediatrician's Exam

Your baby will be checked during the first few days of his life by a pediatrician who will:

- Listen to your baby's heart and lungs

- Feel your baby's abdomen to check whether the organs inside seem the normal size

- Check your baby's reflexes to make sure that his nervous system has developed well

- Test your baby's hips. This is an important test. Some babies have what are called "clicky hips." This means the sockets in the hip bone, which hold the long bones of his legs, are too shallow. Shallow hip sockets may permit the leg bones to slip out. If the baby is not treated for this condition, he will have trouble crawling and walking. But if clicky hips are noticed soon after the baby's birth, they can be treated.

With treatment, the sockets of the hips deepen and keep the long bones in place. The treatment involves putting the baby in double diapers to keep his legs wide apart. Or a plastic "frog splint" over his diaper can be used, which is designed to hold his legs apart. The baby needs to wear double diapers or the splint for a few weeks. In most cases, the problem is solved by then. A small number of babies will need an operation when they are one or two years old.

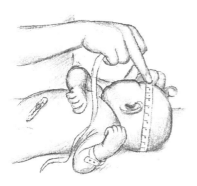

Measuring the baby's head

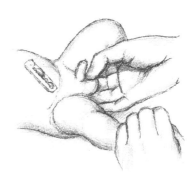

Checking the baby's genitals

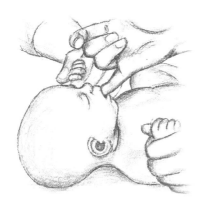

Checking the baby's palate

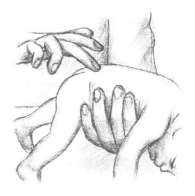

Checking the spine and back passage

The First 24 Hours

Women react in very different ways after labor. Some feel exhausted and want nothing except to sleep. Others are very alert and can't sleep:

"When I had him, I couldn't sleep the first night at all. I was awake most of the night just looking at him. His face was toward me. I couldn't quite believe what had happened."

"I felt calm and had lots of sleep."

Both types of reactions are completely normal. Wanting to be left alone to sleep after your labor is over does not make you a bad mother. If you can't sleep and want to spend all your time looking at your baby, that's fine too. Some babies seem to need frequent feeding in the first 24 hours after birth. Others are too busy looking at the new world. They seem too excited to nurse.

"The baby slept all night. But she hasn't done it since."

"She didn't sleep very much during the first day. I think she was as excited as I was."

"Tom didn't nurse much during the first 24 hours. I felt like he was getting over the birth and he was letting me do the same. He didn't really wake me very much."

"He nursed a lot during the first 24 hours."

Newborn babies need very little milk in the first day of life. If your baby goes to the breast only a couple of times or has only two or three bottles, there's no need to worry.

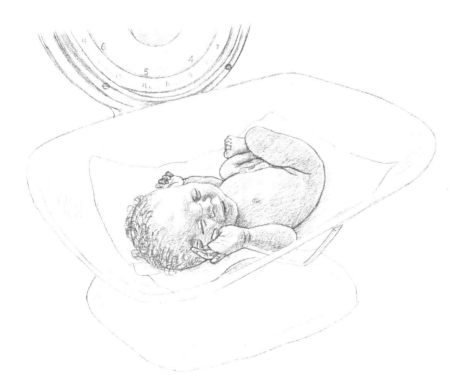

How Long to Stay in the Hospital

Some women find comfort in spending a couple of days in the hospital after the birth. They feel secure knowing there is always a doctor or nurse on hand if there is a problem with the baby. Others find hospitals stressful. Their choice is to go home as quickly as possible: *"I went home 20 hours after I'd had the baby. I didn't want to stay any longer. The staff that was trying to help me breast-feed were always touching, always bothering me. Plus they gave me conflicting advice."*

Conflicting advice is less likely if the woman is cared for by a midwife or a couple of midwives whom she knows: *"During 36 hours in the hospital, I must have had four different nurses show me how to nurse the baby."*

The support the woman receives during the first days and weeks with her new baby is vital. If she is in the hospital after the birth, the hospital staff can affect her a great deal. Their attitude can make all the difference between her feeling strong enough to cope with a new lifestyle and feeling very insecure:

> ## The Apgar Score
> ### (named after Dr. Virginia Apgar)
>
> After your baby has been born and given to you to hold, the doctor or midwife will make a quick check of how healthy he is. She does this by noting his:
> – Color
> – Heart rate
> – Breathing
> – Movements
> – Reflexes
>
> and giving him a score of 0, 1 or 2 for each of these. Your baby is given an Apgar score one minute after his birth and again five minutes later. He might have a score of 7 at one minute. Then, as his breathing becomes stronger and his color changes from blue-purple to pink, a score of 10 at five minutes. If the Apgar score is low at one minute or at five minutes, the nurse will call a doctor to look at your baby and see if he needs special help.

"One day, the nurse told me off for holding my baby. She told me to wheel him around. She said I was not supposed to carry the baby. That really upset me. I didn't know what the right thing to do was."

"It hit me hard the first couple of days! Here was the baby—with me for the rest of my life. But the support I had from the hospital was very good. The nurses were great—very patient."

Some women really enjoy being with other new mothers in the hospital. They find their company supportive. But other women long for the privacy of their own homes: *"I was glad to be at home with my stitches and leaking breasts. It was nice to be in my own bathroom."*

Your Baby's First Feeding

If you want to breast-feed your baby, put him to the breast as soon as he is born. Newborn babies are often very alert. They may remain wide awake for quite a few hours. Make the most of this time and his interest in the world. Start to learn with him about breast-feeding.

The most important thing to get right is the position of your baby on the breast. Ask your midwife to help you. If you make sure he takes your breast properly right from the start, you won't get sore nipples. He is likely to feel much more content if he can fill his stomach well.

Don't worry if your baby doesn't seem to nurse too much, or doesn't seem to get the hang of breast-feeding at all. There's plenty of time for you both to learn. Babies don't need many feedings in the first 24 hours of their lives. They often spend many of those hours sleeping. Some will only want to go to the breast two or three times in the day. That's quite normal. It's also quite normal if your baby wants to nurse much more often.

The first kind of milk your baby receives from you is called *colostrum*. Colostrum contains antibodies to all sorts of diseases. Colostrum gives your baby a great start in life, but there isn't much of it. Don't worry! Your baby won't starve while he waits for you to make more milk. Nature has made sure that he has built up plenty of fat stores during the final weeks in your uterus. These will keep him going until your mature milk starts to come in after a few days.

Breast-fed babies don't need anything except breast milk. They don't need water. They don't need formula milk. They just need you!

Being with other women in the hospital may not be pleasant if you are the only one bottle-feeding or the only one breast-feeding: *"The other mothers had their bottles. I couldn't relax. Each time I breast-fed, someone pulled the curtains around me."*

Sometimes women hear of news stories about babies being stolen from hospitals. These stories may also cause some women to take their babies to the safety of their own homes as soon as they can: *"While I was in the hospital, I used to sleep with the baby in bed with me. I worried all the time that she might be stolen."*

How long a woman wants to stay in the hospital should be her own choice. In the United States, health plans are now required to let new mothers stay in the hospital for at least two days after a vaginal birth, if they choose. They can stay four days after a Cesarean section. A longer stay would cost the mother more. In Canada, the stay is about 2-1/2 days after a vaginal birth, and nearly four days after a C-section.

Babies Who Need Special Care

Some babies need to be cared for in the neonatal intensive care unit (NICU) after they are born. Babies may need special care when:

- They have been born too soon; that is, before 37 weeks of pregnancy
- They are very small, even if they have been in the uterus for more than 37 weeks
- They have had a hard time during labor. They are twins or triplets or more
- They are born with a problem with a major organ, such as the heart or kidneys
- They have been born with a problem such as Down syndrome
- They are having problems breathing

What you can do if your baby is in the intensive care unit

- Stroke your baby. Hold his hand. Touch him. If you are allowed to, give him lots of cuddles.

Babies who are ill at birth may need to have a lot of unpleasant things done to them. They may need to have IV drips put in their hands or head. They may need a tube passed through their nose down into their stomach. They may need to have blood samples taken. They may need a tube put into their lungs to help them breathe. Even when done gently, these things can upset the baby. He will need your comfort afterward. Sick babies' feelings matter as much as their bodies do. And so do yours! You need to hold your baby as much as possible, and he needs you to hold him.

- Express breast milk for your baby. A nurse will show you how to use a breast pump. Your milk can be given to your baby down a tube, if that is how he is being fed. Learn how to tube-feed your baby yourself.
- Wash your baby and change his diapers.
- Ask if you can stay in the hospital while your baby is in the intensive care unit. Some hospitals have rooms for parents whose babies are sick.
- Talk to the nurses and doctors. Ask them to explain your baby's treatment. Ask again if you don't understand something. Say that you want an honest account of your baby's condition.
- When you phone the intensive care unit, ask to speak to the nurse who cares for your baby.
- Take lots of photos of your baby. Most new parents are eager to start an album right away. There's no reason why you shouldn't, too. You also have a baby.
- Put some small toys you have chosen for your baby in his crib.
- When your baby can be dressed, dress him in the clothes you have bought for him. Even if they're much too big, they're his. Wearing them will help you to see him as your baby rather than the hospital's.
- Ask for help at home—from your mother, mother-in-law, sister, relatives, friends. Ask people who will simply help you cope without making any demands on you.

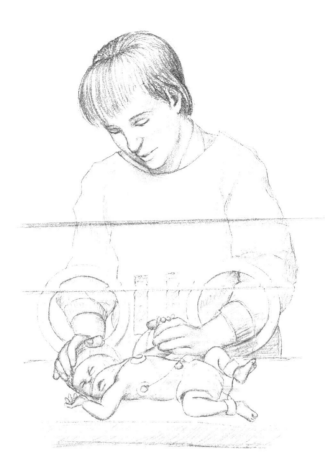

However, in Canada the length of stay may be different depending on the hospital, territory or province.

Women who are very nervous about their new duties will, if they are not rushed, slowly grow in confidence. Soon they will be ready and happy to go home: *"I stayed in the hospital five days. The first few days I didn't want to go home. I thought I would never cope. By the end I was ready to go home, happy to go home."*

Bringing Your Baby Home

Even when the woman has decided to go home, leaving the hospital can take a lot of courage: *"I'd been in the hospital for almost a week. I said, 'I'm doing fine. I want to go home.' But once I was in the car and going home, I felt panicky because now I was on my own. This was it."*

Often, the person who provides the comfort the mother needs most is her baby: *"I was scared to leave the hospital. I thought, 'There are so many things I don't know how to do. I don't know how to breast-feed.' I was sure something awful would happen as soon as I got home. It helped that the baby nursed really well just after I got back. I started to think, 'Maybe it's all right.'"*

The worry women feel about bringing the baby home is often balanced by immense pride and excitement. The house takes on a new feeling. Now it is home for one more person:

"I took her on a tour when we got home. I showed her the kitchen and her bedroom. It was just lovely."

"The first night at home, I just lay there. I felt so excited. I was practically sick with excitement because it was something so new and so wonderful."

Once you're home, away from healthcare providers, small worries can become huge ones:

"I never knew babies could make so much noise at night. Babies grunt when they breathe. That really worried me."

Expressing Breast Milk for Your Baby in Intensive Care

An electric breast pump is the most efficient way to express milk. You will be able to use a pump at the hospital while you are there. You may be able to borrow one to take home if you leave the hospital before your baby. If you can't borrow a pump from the hospital, you should be able to rent one from either:

- La Leche League
  1-800-LA-LECHE
  (847) 519-7730

- La Leche League Canada
  (613) 448-1842

or

- Medela, Inc.
  1-800-TELL-YOU

- With an electric pump, you can pump both breasts at the same time. This will help build up your milk supply as quickly as possible.

- Expect to pump very little milk at first. The amount you collect will increase slowly with regular pumping.

- Take advice from the nurses in the intensive care unit about how often to pump and for how long.

- Your expressed milk can be fed to your baby through the tube in his nose. When he becomes stronger, he will no longer accept the tube. But he still may not be ready to be fully breast-fed. During this time you can feed him your expressed milk from a tiny cup designed for small or sick babies. It's better not to give your baby a bottle if you plan to breast-feed. Bottle-fed babies nurse from a nipple in a very different way from breast-fed babies.

"He slept very well on the first night home. He would have slept better if I hadn't kept poking him just to make sure he was still breathing."

It is normal for new parents to be very anxious about their baby's health and safety. There's probably no way around it: Anxiety is a natural process that ensures babies are well cared for when they are just getting started in life. When new mothers worry, they ask for help and begin to learn from others with more experience. This is one way they can gain knowledge about baby care. In time they will learn to feel secure about themselves as mothers:

"I was panicky about how hot he was. I got out this booklet about SIDS and called my mother. I said, 'I don't know how hot he should be!' I was panicky. She calmed me down."

Coping with Visitors

Some women love being at the center of attention when they come home from the hospital. They feel on top of the world, with no worries about coping. They enjoy showing off their baby to as many people as possible: *"I found all of it so much fun. Friends called all the time and I had tons of visitors. It was like one long party. We saw all our friends, and I really enjoyed that. It didn't seem intrusive. It helped me get back to normal."*

But others need more time to get over the birth. They need to be quiet and get used to being a new family: *"I just wanted the three of us to be together."*

Other people's help is not always a blessing. Help in the early days often comes from those nearest to you: your partner, your own parents and your in-laws. All of them are busy getting used to their new roles as a father or as grandparents. They may feel unsure about what to do and what not to do for you. They may worry about caring for the baby in a way you don't like much. Some people know just how to help without making a fuss or making you feel obliged to them. Others end up making more work for you than you had before: *"When I got home, my mother-in-law was there. I could have done without that, to be honest. I just felt so tired. I would have liked time to unpack my bag and get cleaned up and things like that. I felt very tired. I thought to myself, 'This isn't right!' I was glad when she left."*

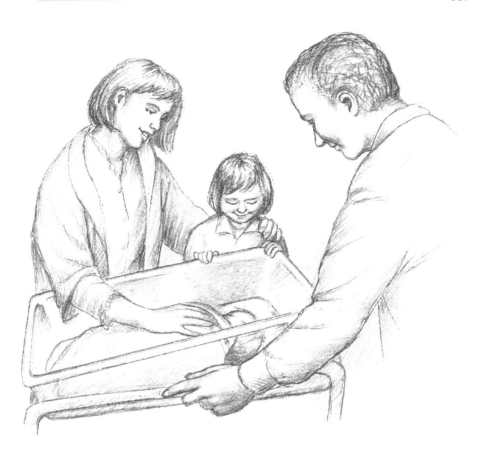

The best kind of support comes from someone who will simply do the household chores and let you spend time with the baby: *"My mother-in-law came from Massachusetts. I don't know what I would have done without her. She made sure the laundry basket wasn't overflowing, cleaned the toilet, and made sure I ate regularly. She made endless, endless cups of tea. I did nothing except look after the baby."*

It is more common today than it used to be for partners to get involved in baby care. Some men are eager to share the day-to-day routines as soon as possible: *"My boyfriend couldn't stop bathing Guy. Each time he had a poopy diaper, he'd say, 'Oh, he'd better have a bath.' He'd give him a bath, and I just let him do it because that was what he enjoyed doing."*

Being able to accept help from your partner means that you have time for yourself. Watching him playing with the baby can be very special: *"I think men used to be deprived. It seems like it's much easier for them*

Tests Your Baby Will Have in the First Days of Life

Genetic Screening

A day or two after the birth, your baby will have a few drops of blood drawn from his heel. You may find this much more painful than your baby does. He is likely to cry a great deal, but it is worthwhile. Your baby's blood will checked for:

- *Phenylketonuria*—when the baby can't break down the protein in his food properly. The half-way broken-down products are toxic. They can gather in the brain and cause brain damage.

- *Galactosemia*—when the baby can't digest sugar properly. He may also have problems with his sight, his liver, kidneys and brain.

- *Hypothyroidism*—when the baby has too little thyroid hormone. The baby will become brain damaged.

Be reassured that these conditions do *not* mean the baby is brain damaged at birth. But babies with these conditions will become so if they are not treated. Genetic screening helps healthcare providers diagnose these conditions. Then they can start treating a baby who is affected as soon as possible. A baby treated for phenylketonuria, galactosemia or hypothyroidism from the early days of his life will thrive. He can grow up and become a normal intelligent adult.

Blood Tests for Jaundice

A day or so after birth, the skin of some babies becomes somewhat yellow. They can look almost as if they have a suntan. This means they have jaundice. It is common for babies to become slightly jaundiced. In the uterus, they have a large number of red blood cells to carry oxygen around their bodies. After they are born, they don't need as many red blood cells and start to break down some of them. The broken-down red blood cells are passed in the baby's urine. If this process doesn't happen quickly enough, they remain in the body and stain the skin yellow. In most cases, the best way to get rid of jaundice is to feed your baby as often as you can. Breast-fed babies don't need to be given bottles to increase their intake of milk. They just need to be put to the breast more often.

By the seventh day of the baby's life, any sign of jaundice is nearly always gone. A few babies have severe jaundice. They will have their blood checked to see if they need phototherapy to help them. This means laying the baby, naked except for a bandage to protect his eyes, beneath a blue light. It is hard for mothers whose babies need phototherapy treatment. They must be kept apart from their babies in the very early days, just when cuddling them feels so important. But phototherapy is often only given for a day or two. And you can, of course, take your baby out from under the light and hold him while you nurse him.

Vitamin K

You need vitamin K so your blood will clot properly. Newborn babies have very little of it. A small number of newborns suffer from bleeding problems in the first few days or weeks of their lives. To protect these few, it has become the custom to give vitamin K to all babies at birth. In the past, it was most often given as a shot.

Recent research has shown that babies who were given a shot of vitamin K at birth may be at increased risk of getting cancer in childhood compared to babies who were not given vitamin K, or who were given it by mouth. Other studies have not found such a link.

It is hard to know what to do now. To be on the safe side, if your baby is to receive vitamin K, you may want to ask that it be given by mouth, instead of as a shot. The trouble with this is that vitamin K is not made to be given by mouth. Babies get the vitamin K that is meant to be given as a shot.

Breast-fed babies have extra-low levels of vitamin K. No one knows why. This could put them at greater risk of having a bleeding problem. But it may be that their low level of vitamin K protects them from something we don't know about yet.

Ask your doctor or midwife about vitamin K. You may want to make your own choice about giving vitamin K to your baby. Discuss it with your doctor or midwife before your baby is born.

now just to be with their babies. It's really nice to watch Ross and Lisa together. Besides, it gives me a break!"

Some women find it is hard to let their partners care for the baby and learn by making their own mistakes: *"Matt was really good. He used to take Owen away when he was crying at night. But I would get really wound up about the way he looked after him. It wasn't my way—or the way I wanted him to do it. It was stupid, I guess, that I got so tense. All he was doing was trying to relieve me of worry."*

"I got really sick. I panicked when I thought my husband was going to look after Angie."

Keep in touch with each other's feelings by talking. If you can, enjoy some time together away from the baby. This can help resolve upsets. When a couple works as a team, the burden of caring for a new baby seems much lighter: *"I wasn't worried. I thought I could cope. Russell and I did things together."*

Postpartum Exercise and Support Groups

Postpartum exercise classes have become popular. They are designed to ensure that you get your body back into shape safely. Classes are run by:

- Hospitals
- Fitness centers

You may have to pay a fee for these classes. But if you can't afford it, say so. You may be able to get a discount.

Your Body after Your Baby Is Born

In our culture, women don't expect to feel sick after giving birth to a baby. They expect to take labor in stride and be back to normal quickly. But even a strong, healthy woman can feel shaky after she has had a baby. Give yourself enough time to recover: *"I was amazed at how long it took my body to recover after labor. On the second night, the baby wouldn't settle down for two or three hours. I tried to carry him around but my legs felt like jelly. I was shocked at how weak I was."*

"The staircase was like a mountain. I had to rest every two or three steps. Then I crawled along the hall to the bedroom."

It often takes a long time to recover from a Cesarean section. Some mothers, though, are up and around pretty quickly: *"I was given good pain relief in the hospital. I came home after six days. My incision healed fully within a week of the birth. I haven't had any pain since leaving the hospital, either. In fact, it's hard to believe I had major abdominal surgery."*

Other women take much longer to recover than this. It's not a question of strength of spirit. It's just that each person's response to surgery is different:

"The first time you sit up after a C-section, it feels like you're on fire. You have to pull yourself up with your arms. And when you have to stand up the first time, you can't stand up straight because of your incision. You tend to bend over to prevent pulling on your stitches. It took me at least six weeks to feel normal again. It was about nine months before the final twinges of pain from the incision had gone."

A woman who has had a Cesarean needs help when she gets home. Try to find someone to help you. If you can, ask a family member or friend to stay with you and relieve you of day-to-day chores. You will probably recover much faster.

The changes in your body that happened during nine months of pregnancy take a while to be reversed. For instance, it's normal to have a very heavy vaginal flow after giving birth. This is a mixture of blood and mucus and is called *lochia*. It is much heavier than a period and lasts two to six weeks: *"Be prepared for a lot of blood for the first couple of days. Buy giant, hospital-size pads. It took six weeks for my blood loss to stop completely."*

If you have had a lot of stitches in your perineum or a lot of bruising, it may be a while before you can sit in comfort: *"I was bruised but I didn't have stitches. It was no fun to sit down, but not so bad going to the bathroom. If I sat down too long and then stood up, blood rushed to the sore parts. That hurt!"*

Some women have severe afterbirth pains. They are not common with a first baby, but fairly common with subsequent babies. The uterus continues to contract at intervals for a few days after labor is over.

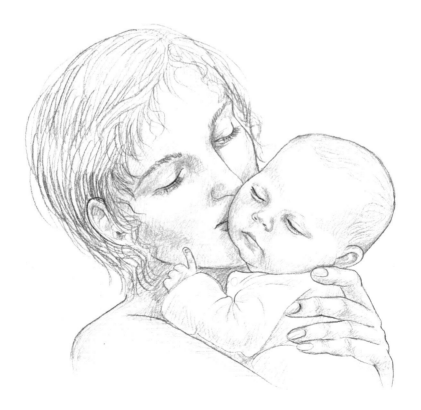

Your Body after Your Baby Is Born

After your baby is born, your body has to get back to the way it was before you became pregnant. You can do a number of things for yourself in the first few days after giving birth that will help.

- Get up and around as soon as you can. This helps you in all sorts of ways:

  – You are in better spirits if you don't lie in bed all day.

  – You prevent blood from pooling in your legs. This can make you prone to varicose veins or to getting clots in your veins. (Clots in your veins can be dangerous!)

  – You help your uterus to empty properly. After giving birth, you will have a heavy discharge, like a period. It's called *lochia* and changes from red to pink to whitish-brown over the next two or three weeks. You may also find that you pass some blood clots in the first days after the birth. This is normal, but your doctor or midwife will still want to know what they were like. Show them to her, if you can.

  – You can urinate more easily. Some women find it hard to pee after they've had a baby. Their bladder has been bruised during the birth. It's much easier to pee on a toilet in private than on a bedpan in a hospital bed!

- *Enjoy a good diet.* Lots of women are slightly or very anemic after giving birth (not enough iron). You can help get your strength back if you choose to eat foods rich in iron such as green leafy vegetables and red meat. Vitamin C helps your body absorb the iron in your diet, so plenty of fresh fruit also helps. Choose foods that are rich in fiber to help your bowels. Eat potatoes with their skins on, whole-grain bread, cereals with bran and unpeeled fruit.

- *Exercise your pelvic floor* several times a day. If you have stitches in your perineum, the exercise will help you heal more quickly. The exercise ensures a good supply of blood to this area.

- *Ask for help.* The early days with a new baby can be exhausting. Accept help from those who offer it. In many cultures, women have no household duties for several weeks after the birth of their babies.

- *Rest*—easier said than done! You have to be strict with yourself so that when the baby is asleep, you relax. Don't worry if you can't get to sleep—just take the phone off the hook. Watch TV, read, have something to eat or close your eyes.

Putting the baby to the breast often stimulates afterpains. That's because the hormone that lets down milk from the breasts also makes the uterus contract:

"The second time around, for the first few days it was like having periods cramps each time I put her to the breast. I noticed it a little after the first birth. But it was much worse the second time."

Some women, perhaps not many, have no problems at all after their babies are born. They bounce back to health right away: *"I didn't have any problems. I was fatter when I was pregnant with Alexandra than I had ever been before. I think it carried over. I did get very tired about two weeks after she was born. But then I went to stay with my mom for a few days, and I was fine. I have to admit I was surprised. I thought I would be dragging around for weeks feeling tired and sore."*

Your Emotions after Your Baby Is Born

No one has fully explained why so many women have what are called the *baby blues* a few days after the birth of their babies. In hospitals you can sometimes find a ward full of women crying their hearts out. The nurse explains that they're all new mothers, and they've gotten the blues together! A number of things may contribute to getting the blues: Hormone levels are changing. Fatigue from the ordeal of labor can combine with tiredness from lack of sleep. Mothers also begin to realize on a deep level that life will never be the same again. Often, a very small thing will trigger a flood of tears:

"I woke up at night and I thought, 'What if there's a Third World War, and we're all blown up in a nuclear explosion? How could I have brought a baby into this world?' I felt so bad! I went through a box and a half of tissues before Carl arrived the next morning."

"I was in the hospital by myself, crying and thinking, 'I've got a baby. What am I going to do!'"

"I sobbed my heart out by the refrigerator. Andy offered to do the shopping. I gave him a list. He didn't buy any of the things I wanted. They were all the wrong brands. I didn't have anything I needed. I just sat down with the refrigerator door open and sobbed. I couldn't help it."

Your confidence in being a mother will be boosted by having people around you who don't criticize you. They should let you care for your baby in your own way: *"My mother came for an extended visit when I left the hospital. I don't know what I would have done without her. Not that she did much, but she was a comforting presence. She didn't look after the baby. She let me do that and often told me what a really good job I was doing. Her saying that meant a lot."*

Feeling Depressed

Women may feel low in the first weeks and months after having a baby for a number of very good reasons:

- *Changed lifestyle*—You may have decided that your baby will not prevent you from doing all the things you used to do. But then you find that your life does change—a lot. You have to go with what your baby wants rather than the other way around.

- *Changes in relationships*—The people who are important to you will see you in a new way now that you are a mother. Your partner may feel, and you may feel, that you are no longer his friend and lover. It can seem as though your body and energy have been taken over by the baby.

- *Loneliness*—It's easy to get trapped within the four walls of your home when you have a new baby. Going out can be very tricky. You have to take diapers, wipes, a changing mat, sleep suits and perhaps bottles. Staying at home may seem a lot easier. But not seeing anyone for days and not speaking with any adults is almost certain to make you feel low.

- *Tiredness*—Many people become bad-tempered and feel they can't cope with life when they are tired. Most new mothers are very, very tired during the first weeks, months and sometimes years of their babies' lives.

Getting Out of the House

- Decide that you will go out.
- Give yourself plenty of time to get things ready. Bring two spare diapers, a plastic bag to put dirty diapers in and diaper wipes. You may want a clean sleep suit, tissues, a bottle of formula if you're bottle-feeding, or breast pads if you're breast-feeding. You'll need a large bag to carry everything in.
- If you can, try to feed your baby about an hour before you go out. Then change her so that she's settled.
- Make sure you've also made time to go to the bathroom, brush your hair and put on some make-up, if you wear it. You need to feel confident to meet other people.
- Go out!

The baby blues can last for a few hours or a few days, but they nearly always pass:

"I was fine until about two days after I came home. Then I got very depressed. I went from being high to being depressed. But it didn't last long, a couple of days."

If your baby blues go on for weeks and weeks, you may have a more serious depression. Talk to your doctor about it. If you can't face seeing a healthcare provider, at least talk to *someone* about how you feel. There are good counseling services now to help women who suffer from postpartum depression.

Meeting Other Mothers

Having a baby gives you a great chance to make new friends. It demands a certain amount of effort on your part. But it's worth it. The friends you make will help you learn about all the things you need to know as a parent:

- Tips for soothing crying babies
- Which shops are the best for baby things
- How to amuse a toddler indoors on a rainy day
- Coping with children who are picky eaters
- How good the local play groups are, and so on

Your local library can be a good place to find out about Mother and Baby/Toddler Groups that meet near you.

Look for signs in baby-store windows, at preschools and at your pediatrician's office. Ask other moms. They'll be sure to know. Groups are run by:

- Health centers. Some offer post-partum courses with the opportunity to discuss the joys and worries of early parenthood.

  Cost: May be free

- Local churches or temples. You may not have to be a member to attend the Mother and Toddler Group.

  Cost: a small sum or may be free

- Community Centers

  Cost: a small sum or may be free

Feelings after a Cesarean

After a Cesarean, some women need to come to terms with the fact that their baby wasn't born the way they had planned it, without intervention. They also have to deal with an altered body image. Many mothers feel content with the decision to have a Cesarean. They recognize that going through major surgery in order to give birth is not an easy option. But others are upset with themselves. They feel that not being able to have a vaginal birth is a failure: *"I had a lot of strong emotions afterward. I felt like a failure as a mother for not being able to give birth 'properly.' I felt guilty that I had let down my partner somehow for not having the birth we had planned and discussed."*

The incision is a constant reminder of the way in which the baby was born. Some women find that their low spirits translate into a physical weakness, which can last a long time: *"I hate my stomach. It hangs over the incision. It really affects my body image. It has taken me at least a year to get some of my self-confidence back. I used to be very fit and strong. But I'm only now beginning to think, 'Yes, I can do that.'"*

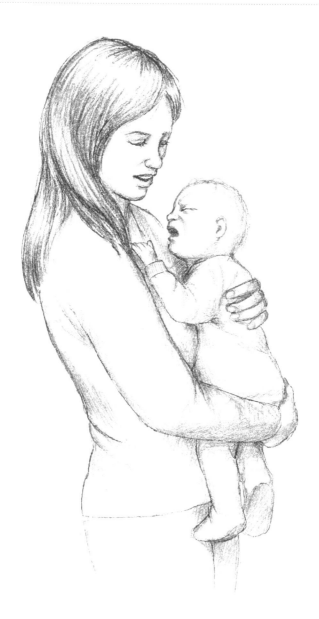

Getting over emotional trauma requires support. You need to be able to rely on people who will simply listen to your story and try to understand your feelings, without making judgments. It helps to think about whether you have a friend like this who is good at listening. Or perhaps you know of someone who has been through the same type of experience. If not, call Sidelines (see "Useful Addresses") for referral to someone who has had a Cesarean and felt upset about it afterward:

"The best thing was a friend who'd also had an emergency C-section. She talked frankly with me about how I felt."

"For me, coming to terms with everything that happened was helped, first, by going through my chart. I needed to put together what happened. Then I talked again and again about the C-section to Walt. He was great and coped really well, although he says he was in shock for a long time."

"What helped me get over what happened was joining a Cesarean support group. Helping other women get through the tough times helped me heal my own hurt."

Feelings about Your Baby

Some women's feelings for their baby are immensely strong from the moment of birth: *"My love for my baby was so amazing! I wanted another baby right away! And my friend who came to see me in the hospital says my first words were, 'I'll have to do this again! It's fantastic!'"*

They have an intense need to protect the baby and keep him close at all times: *"I held him the whole time. I didn't want to put him in the crib at the hospital. The nurse said, 'You need some rest now.' I watched her put him in the crib and go out the door. Then I just picked him up again."*

As adults, we know that some couples fall in love at first sight. The minute they clap eyes on each other, they are sure they were made to be together. For others, falling in love is a process that takes months and perhaps years. Relationships that start in either way can be strong and good. The fact that you're not a "love at first sight" person doesn't matter. Some women are instantly in love with their babies. Others find their love grows slowly over time:

"I can honestly say I didn't want to take my baby home from the hospital. I wanted to leave him there. Then when I did take him home, I felt nothing for him at all. That lasted for four or five weeks. Now I feel like I am having a passionate love affair with my baby."

"I'd expected a sudden rush when I saw her. It came more slowly than that. It was very powerful, but not there all at once."

Feeding Your Baby

You may feel your most important task, in the first days and weeks of your baby's life, is feeding her properly. The choice whether to bottle-feed or breast-feed is a personal one:

"I can't understand why anyone would want to breast-feed. I see the bottle as a symbol of women's liberation."

"I felt really proud of my little boy, who was still being breast-fed at six months. I thought, 'That's all me. I've done that.'"

The success of either method will depend, in large measure, on how you feel about your decision and the support you have.

No matter how you feed your baby, there will be things you worry about. It seems so important, in those first few weeks, to get the feeding right. Doctors and nurses sometimes seem to measure how good a mother you are by how much weight your baby puts on. If you bottle-feed your baby, you will be anxious about how to sterilize the bottles and prepare them correctly. You may have been shown how to do this by a friend or a nurse in the hospital. If you weren't, follow the instructions on the can of formula or box of sterilizing tablets and you won't go wrong.

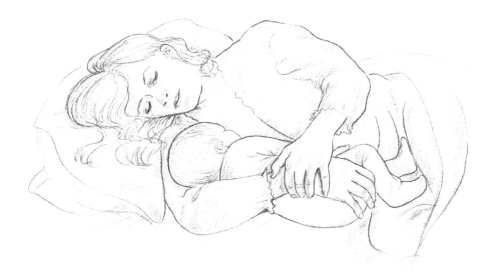

Putting Your Baby to the Breast

- Make sure you are sitting or lying in comfort, with good support for your back.
- Use plenty of cushions or pillows to bring the baby up to the level of your breasts.
- Hold your baby close. Turn her so that her chest faces your chest.
- Make sure her head is in line with her body and not turned to one side.
- Your baby should have her upper lip on a level with your nipple. You can get your baby to open her mouth by rubbing her top lip against your nipple.
- Once her mouth opens *wide,* move her quickly onto the breast. (She should take a lot of the breast into her mouth, not just your nipple. So her mouth needs to be *open very wide.*)
- Relax and enjoy nursing!

Have I got it right?

Check: Are your baby's lips curled back? (You may need a mirror to see this or a friend to tell you.)

Check: Can you can still see some of the areola (the colored skin around your nipple)? More of it should be showing above your baby's top lip than below her bottom lip.

Check: Does it hurt you when your baby nurses? If it does, take her off the breast by slipping your finger into the corner of her mouth, and start again. You may have a strong sensation (*not* a painful one) when your baby first starts nursing. But this should be gone within 5 or 6 seconds.

Check: Does your baby's nursing action seem to be strong and rhythmic?

Can you see her ears wiggling or the muscles in her temples moving? Your baby uses her tongue and lower jaw to do the work of suckling. If her cheeks are moving in and out, she's not nursing properly. You need to take her off the breast and put her back in the right position, with her mouth open wide.

The right way to breast-feed

- The baby nurses from the breast and not from the nipple
- The baby nurses at the breast as often and as long as she wants to
- The baby nurses from the first breast until it is soft and empty and then from the second only if she wants to
- The baby needs nothing except breast milk. She doesn't need formula, and she doesn't need water.

REMEMBER

The more often you nurse your baby, the more milk you will make. Your baby knows just how often to nurse.

All these are normal:

- Your baby nurses eight or ten times a day.
- Your milk looks yellow in the early days and then thin and watery later on.
- Your baby likes to nurse for a long time. Or, your baby nurses very quickly.
- Your baby has a dirty diaper at each feeding.
- Your baby has one dirty diaper a day.
- Your baby has one dirty diaper a week.

While You Are Breast-feeding

Take Care of Yourself

- Eat well and have regular meals. If you don't have time to make meals, have lots of healthy snacks such as sandwiches, cereal, nuts, raisins, fruit, yogurt.

- Drink when you feel thirsty. Water or fruit juice are best. Stay away from drinks with caffeine (coffee, tea, hot chocolate, cola) and alcohol. You don't have to drink milk to make milk, but it can be a useful snack.

- Rest as much as you can. If you eat, drink and rest, you'll make plenty of milk for your baby. And you'll enjoy nursing her.

If You Need Help

If you have a problem with breast-feeding, such as sore nipples, don't struggle with it alone. You can get help from:

- Your midwife or nurse

- A breast-feeding counselor. Many health plans cover the cost of lactation (breast-feeding) counseling. Or contact La Leche League (see "Useful Addresses"). You don't have to be a member to contact one of their counselors. Counselors are there to give free support to any woman who needs it.

Breast-feeding is a different kind of learning process. It involves the baby finding out how he can get the milk from the breast. And it involves the mother finding out how she can nurse her baby in comfort.

Some babies just seem to get the hang of breast-feeding right away: *"I used to get sore, painful breasts each month before my period. I thought it would be like that when I nursed, but it was much better."*

But other women have to work their way through problems such as sore nipples and the worry of not knowing whether the baby has had enough milk: *"I can't wait for the moment when I can just stick her on without having to think about it."*

The first days are often the hardest. It's at this time that a lot of women give up breast-feeding or come close to it: *"I loved my baby. But there were times when I wished I didn't have to be the one to nurse her."*

Being tired can make the effort of learning a new skill seem too great. The attraction of bottle-feeding can be very strong. But women who choose to bottle-feed are not without their depressed moments either: *"I was up to here with sterilizing bottles."*

You become more confident about your chosen method of feeding as your baby grows: *"Only one thing kept me going: Jacob's obvious pleasure in breast-feeding and his bouncing good health."*

You may receive conflicting advice about infant feeding. Try to decide which people make you feel good about your mothering, and listen to them. People who undermine your confidence are of no service to you at all. The supportive ones will help you feel happy and on top of things as a mother: *"Dean was nursing all day. I was sure I didn't have enough milk. But I had a visit from the midwife, and she checked my breasts. She said, 'Don't be silly, you could feed all the babies on the block.' It gave me a real boost."*

Caring for Your Baby

These days it seems that few women have cared for or even held a small baby before they give birth to their own. The daily routine of caring for a new baby can be daunting. Women used to learn about baby care by watching or helping with baby-care tasks from a very early age. Today, many women have to learn how to care for babies by reading books, asking other people and seeing what works:

"The first diaper change took half an hour. It involved two of us running up and down the stairs because all our things were in the wrong places. If someone had filmed this little baby just lying there while these two crazy people ran around the house . . . Well!"

"I just didn't feel confident about holding her. In the end, Fernando said, 'Do you think she should have a bath today?' and we did it together. It was like surgery. We laid out towels all over her bedroom floor. He brought the bath and filled it with water. We'd gotten bubble bath and all the kits that people buy. We didn't use any of it. We just sort of plopped her in and plopped her out again and that was it. I was so worried that she'd get cold."

With second babies, mothers find they are far more relaxed. They are often better able to enjoy the early weeks of their new child's life:

"Second babies are much easier than first babies. I made it hard on myself the first time even though he was a very easy baby. I did everything by the book. I was always washing. Things took so long."

Sleepless Nights

Help the baby get into a routine by being quiet with him at night:

• Don't change him unless he's really wet or dirty.

  – Don't play with him

  – Keep the lighting low

  – Feed him and put him down again right away.

• Discuss with your partner whether it would be good for you to have separate rooms for a while. Then only one person needs to be disturbed for night feedings.

• Or share the night-time feeding and changing. (If you are breast-feeding, pump and save your milk during the day. Then your partner can give the baby your breast milk in a bottle at night.)

• During the day, rest when you can. Try to sleep when the baby sleeps.

• Ask for help during the day so that you can rest.

• The baby will develop a routine, but in his own time, which could take months.

"She'd sleep for six hours, and I'd wonder if something was wrong. I'd worry that babies were not meant to sleep that long! The second time around, you're happy to let them sleep."

After a while, first-time mothers also become more confident in themselves and in their babies: *"You figure out you don't have to be so obsessive, that the baby will survive."*

Lack of Sleep

Most parents are surprised to find how little rest they get during the first weeks of their babies' lives. They also learn how tough it is to be constantly deprived of sleep. Most of us are used to having a sleepless night now and then. But having no sleep for days on end puts people under a strain like nothing else.

Some women learn to deal with broken nights: *"I am surprised that I can keep going day and night, because I'm a person who really likes my sleep. I'm surprised that if she cries in the night, I just think, 'Oh, she's crying,' and I'm happy to go to her. I'm not upset. It doesn't worry me that she's sometimes up all night, and that surprises me."*

For others, the long disturbed nights are very upsetting: *"Beth never let me sleep and I was exhausted. It was a bad time for me. I was so tired."*

"I remember begging the baby for sleep—'Just five minutes, please give me five minutes.' Two hours later, I was still begging him for five minutes."

For the first few weeks of their lives, no babies are likely to be in a "routine." Routines are helpful for small children and adults. But they have no meaning at all to babies: *"I couldn't understand why my baby didn't sleep. She wouldn't settle down until four in the morning. Then she would be awake at six or six-thirty again for another feeding. She never slept at set times. But it is getting better."*

Some women become experts at sleeping whenever they can: *"At night, I'm half-sleeping when I nurse him. I go back to sleep right away when he's finished. If he sleeps during the day, I just stretch out on the couch with a book and fall asleep. I think you have to do that. It's the only way to keep going."*

Sometimes it seems that the pattern of broken nights is a fixed one. The baby may not sleep more than two or three hours without needing you again. In time, most babies do grow into the habit of sleeping for nine or ten hours at night without waking. Hang on to the thought that your small, demanding baby will grow into a little person who learns the difference between day and night: *"It's all a phase. Nothing lasts very long. If it's bad today, a few weeks down the line things will have changed."*

When the Baby Cries and Cries

- Try feeding her (again).
- Then try:
  - Changing her diaper
  - Checking that she is not too warm or too cold
  - Rocking her
  - Holding her
  - Singing to her
  - Playing music to her
  - Holding her and dancing
- Get some support.
- Hand over the baby to your partner, grandparent, sister, relative, friend or next-door neighbor and take a break.
- If the baby is fed, clean and clearly not ill, put her in her crib, shut the door and retreat. Stay away for a fixed period of time (like 10 or 20 minutes). Go to a room where you cannot hear her crying. After—and only after—the fixed time has gone by, go and check her. With any luck, she'll be fast asleep.
- If you're worried at all about the baby's health, call the doctor.
- Call Child Help (1-800-4A-CHILD), a hotline for parents in crisis, some other parents' group, or a friend. It can help to talk to someone who understands what you are going through.
- It's OK to feel angry and upset sometimes. Life with a baby is hard work.

Crying Babies

Many adults cannot take the noise of a baby crying for more than a few minutes. Parents become frantic when they can't stop their babies' crying. A howling baby makes you feel like a poor mother. And there's always the worry at the back of your mind that there may be something wrong. Nine times out of ten, the baby is crying because he is hungry.

But there are times when you feed your baby again and again, change him and cuddle him. And he still goes on crying:

"The baby's crying. You get the milk ready and tell him it's warming up. You give it to him. No, he's still crying, it wasn't that. It must be the diaper. You go upstairs and change the diaper. That doesn't work either— he's still crying. It might be that he's too hot. You check him and put something cooler on. Now he's crying because he's too cold. Perhaps it's gas. By this time, you wonder if he's screaming because he's hungry again."

When their babies cry without stopping, mothers can behave sometimes in ways they never would have thought possible: *"One night, I called for help at two o'clock in the morning. The only nurse I could find said, 'Will you harm your baby?' And I said, 'I'm not going to harm the baby, but I can't stop him crying and I don't want him.' She was very helpful. But if someone had told me that would happen to me, I never would have believed them. I have loved babies for as long as I can remember."*

It's common for babies to have crying spells in the early hours of the evening. The mother is tired at the end of her day. Perhaps her fatigue and stress transmit themselves to the baby. You may never learn why the baby is upset. Once your confidence has grown, you come to accept it as one of those things:

"Often from 7:30 until 9:30 at night, she cries. It seems to be her crying time. After I try to put her down, she gets to the point where she just goes off."

"He's obviously exhausted. But he won't stay in his crib. He's crying because he's so tired. But he still wants to be with us."

Often women are aware that the more uptight they are, the more fretful the baby becomes. Trying to relax can be the answer. But that's often easier said than done! If you can, give the baby to someone else for a while when you're worn out with trying to soothe him. Learning to ask for and to accept help is not easy for many women. But the more support you can get during the early days, months and years of motherhood, the more likely you are to enjoy them: *"If people offer to help, accept it! I should have done that. I was a real martyr. I'd say, 'It's OK, I can manage. I can do ten things at once!' Actually, you can't. Inside, you're falling apart."*

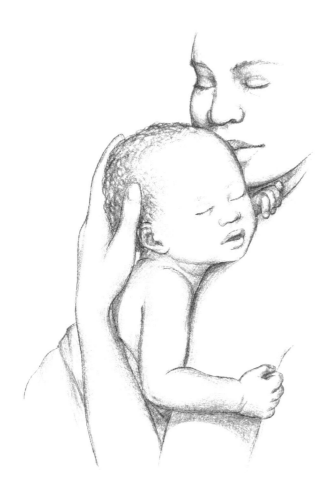

Being a Mother

Some women seem to love being a mother from the word "go:" *"It's great, much easier than I expected."*

It may be more common to find that getting used to your new role takes time. Having a first baby may teach you things about yourself you never knew. It can be hard to find that you're not the sort of person you thought you were: *"I used to work in a nursery with 30 children. I thought I would sail through caring for my own baby. But after a few days of her constant crying, I was running out of patience. I still feel that way, because she cries a lot. Then I get upset with myself for being upset."*

It can be a shock to learn how demanding motherhood is:

"Even if you just want to hang the wash you have to think, 'Where's the baby? What will do I do with her? Will I take her with me or what?'"

"I want to take a shower without having to peep through the curtains and sing all the time just to try and calm down this screaming infant."

Slowly, women grow to understand their own feelings better. They learn what they need to have if they are to be happy as mothers:

"I get very frustrated. I need time with my partner or with my friends. I know I need to have time away from the baby."

"The day came when someone offered to look after the baby for me. I was out the door so fast! The first five minutes of freedom were incredible."

Mothers also become more confident about looking after their babies. They learn to decide for themselves what advice to accept and what to reject:

"They kept telling me to put down the baby. But I simply didn't agree. I hardly put her down until she was crawling. That's what I wanted to do."

Informed Choices

"That's what I wanted to do" nicely sums up the theme of this book. To enjoy being pregnant, giving birth and becoming a mother, you have to make your own decisions. You may listen to the advice of health-care providers and other parents. But in the end you must decide for yourself what you want to do. You can learn from others, but then you have to apply what they say to your own life. And *you* are the only expert about that. Your baby is uniquely yours. You know more about him than anyone else. And your instinct as to what he needs and what you need in order to care for him will almost always be your best guide.

Useful Addresses

General Information

American College of Obstetricians and Gynecologists
 Information about pregnancy, labor, birth or postpartum issues
Resource Center
PO Box 96920
Washington, DC 20090-6920

Family Service Canada
600-220 Laurier Ave.
West Ottawa, Ont. K1P 5Z9
Tel: (613) 230-9960

March of Dimes Birth Defects Foundation
National Office
1275 Mamaroneck Ave.
White Plains, NY 10605

Help for Mother

American Cancer Society
 Help to quit smoking; check your phone book for a local affiliate
Tel. (toll-free): 1-800-227-2345

American Lung Association
 Help to quit smoking; check your phone book for a local affiliate
Tel. (toll-free): 1-800-LUNG USA

W.I.C. Program
 Supplemental Feeding Program for Women, Infants and Children
 In the United States, contact your state or local Department of Public Health

Conception, Pregnancy and Childbirth

American Academy of Husband-Coached Childbirth (Bradley Method)
 Childbirth-educator referrals
PO Box 5224
Sherman Oaks, CA 91413
Tel. (toll-free): (800) 423-2397

American College of Nurse-Midwives
 Information and referral
818 Connecticut Ave. NW
Suite 900
Washington, DC 20006
Tel: (202) 728-9860

American Society for Psycho-prophylaxis in Obstetrics (ASPO/Lamaze)
1200 19th Street NW
Suite 300
Washington, DC 20036-2422
Tel. (toll-free): (800) 368-4404

Association of Labor Assistants and Childbirth Educators (ALACE)
 Provides information and referral
PO Box 38724
Cambridge, MA 02238-2724
Tel: (617) 441-2500

Doulas of North America
1100 23rd Avenue East
Seattle, WA 98112
Fax: (206) 325-0472

Informed Home Birth
Tel: (313) 662-6857

International Cesarean Awareness
Network (ICAN)
1304 Kingsdale Road
Redondo Beach, CA 90278
Tel: (310) 542-6400

International Childbirth
Education Association
PO Box 20048
Minneapolis, MN 55420
Tel: (612) 854-8660

Midwives Alliance of North
America (MANA)
PO Box 175
Newton, KS 67115
Tel: (316) 283-4543

National Association of
Childbearing Centers (NACC)
(Referral to birth centers)
3123 Gottschall Road
Perkiomenville, PA 18074
Tel: (215) 234-8068

Public Citizen's Health
Research Group
 Information about C-sections,
 vaginal births after Cesarean
 [VBAC], other pregnancy-,
 birth-related concerns
1600 20th Street NW
Washington, DC 20009
Tel: (202) 588-1000

After the Birth

Child Help
 Child abuse hotline for parents
 in crisis or children at risk
Tel. (toll-free): (800) 422-4453
(1-800-4A-CHILD)

Depression After Delivery
PO Box 1282
Morrisville, PA 19067
Tel. (toll-free): (800) 944-4773

INFACT Canada
 Provides breast-feeding
 information, support, referral
10 Trinity Square
Toronto, Ont. M5G 1B1
Tel: (416) 595-9819

International Lactation Consultant
Association (ILCA)
200 N. Michigan Ave.
Suite 300
Chicago, IL 60601-3821
Tel: (312) 541-1710

La Leche League Canada
PO Box 29
Chesterville, Ont. K0C 1H0
Tel: (613) 448-1842

La Leche League Canada Français
874 Ville de St. Laurent
Quebec H4L 4W3
Tel: (514) 747-9127

La Leche League International
1400 N. Meacham Rd.
Schaumburg, IL 60173
Tel: (847) 519-7730;
(800) LA-LECHE

Medela, Inc.
 Information, referral for breast
 pumps, breast-feeding
 specialists
PO Box 660
McHenry, IL 60051
Tel. (toll-free): (800) TELL-YOU

Special Situations

About Face Canada
  Information and support for
  parents of a child with a
  cleft palate or other facial
  abnormality
Tel. (toll-free): (800) 665-FACE

About Face U.S.A.
Tel. (toll-free): (800) 225-FACE

CARESS
  Information for parents of
  children with disabilities
PO Box 1492
Washington, DC 20013

Direct Link for the Disabled, Inc.
  Rare disorders, complicated
  situations and denial of
  benefits
PO Box 1036
Solvang, CA 93464
Tel: (805) 688-1603

ECMO Moms and Dads
  Information for parents of
  premature babies
c/o Blair and Gayle Wilson
PO Box 53848
Lubbock, TX 79453
Tel: (806) 794-0259

National Organization for Rare
Disorders (NORD)
PO Box 8923
New Fairfield, CT 06812

National Down Syndrome Society
(NDSS)
666 Broadway
New York, NY 10012-2317
Tel. (toll-free): (800) 221-4602

Sidelines
  For women experiencing a
  complicated pregnancy
  Candace Hurley, executive
  director: (714) 497-2265
  Tracy Hoogenboom:
  (909) 563-6199

If Your Baby Dies

Center for Loss in Multiple Birth
c/o Jean Kollantai
PO Box 1064
Palmer, AK 99645
Tel: (907) 746-6123

Pregnancy and Infant Loss Center
  Information on perinatal
  bereavement
1421 E. Wayzata Blvd.
Suite 30
Wayzata, MN 55391
Tel: (612) 473-9372

SHARE
  Support by telephone and mail
  after bereavement; listing of
  support groups worldwide;
  newsletter
St. Joseph's Health Center
300 First Capitol Drive
St. Charles, MO 63301-2893
Tel. (toll-free): (800) 821-6819

Index